WITHDRAWN

Healing Wounds, Healthy Skin

Yale University Press Health & Wellness

A Yale University Press Health & Wellness book is an authoritative, accessible source of information on a health-related topic. It may provide guidance to help you lead a healthy life, examine your treatment options for a specific condition or disease, situate a healthcare issue in the context of your life as a whole, or address questions or concerns that linger after visits to your healthcare provider.

Joseph A. Abboud, M.D., and Soo Kim Abboud, M.D.,
No More Joint Pain

Thomas E. Brown, Ph.D.,
Attention Deficit Disorder: The Unfocused Mind in Children and Adults

Patrick Conlon,
The Essential Hospital Handbook:
How to Be an Effective Partner in a Loved One's Care

Richard C. Frank, M.D.,
Fighting Cancer with Knowledge and Hope:
A Guide for Patients, Families, and Health Care Providers

Michelle A. Gourdine, M.D.,
Reclaiming Our Health: A Guide to African American Wellness

Marjorie Greenfield, M.D.,
The Working Woman's Pregnancy Book

Ruth H. Grobstein, M.D., Ph.D.,
The Breast Cancer Book: What You Need to Know to Make Informed Decisions

James W. Hicks, M.D.,
Fifty Signs of Mental Illness: A Guide to Understanding Mental Health

Steven L. Maskin, M.D.,
Reversing Dry Eye Syndrome:
Practical Ways to Improve Your Comfort, Vision, and Appearance

Mary Jane Minkin, M.D., and Carol V. Wright, Ph.D.,
A Woman's Guide to Menopause and Perimenopause

Mary Jane Minkin, M.D., and Carol V. Wright, Ph.D.,
A Woman's Guide to Sexual Health

Arthur W. Perry, M.D., F.A.C.S.,
Straight Talk about Cosmetic Surgery

Catherine M. Poole, with DuPont Guerry IV, M.D.,
Melanoma: Prevention, Detection, and Treatment, 2nd ed.

Madhuri Reddy, M.D., M.Sc., and Rebecca Cottrill, R.N., M.Sc.C.H.,
Healing Wounds, Healthy Skin:
A Practical Guide for Patients with Chronic Wounds

E. Fuller Torrey, M.D.,
Surviving Prostate Cancer: What You Need to Know to Make Informed Decisions

Barry L. Zaret, M.D., and Genell J. Subak-Sharpe, M.S.,
Heart Care for Life: Developing the Program That Works Best for You

Healing Wounds, Healthy Skin

*A Practical Guide for Patients
with Chronic Wounds*

Madhuri Reddy, M.D., M.Sc.
Rebecca Cottrill, R.N., M.Sc.C.H.

Illustrations by Victoria Cansino, M.Sc.B.M.C.

Yale UNIVERSITY PRESS
New Haven and London

MEMORIAL LIBRARY
500 N. DUNTON
ARLINGTON HEIGHTS, IL 60004

The information and suggestions contained in this book are not intended to replace the services of your physician or caregiver. Because each person and each medical situation is unique, you should consult your own physician to get answers to your personal questions, to evaluate any symptoms you may have, or to receive suggestions for appropriate medications.

The authors have attempted to make this book as accurate and up to date as possible, but it may nevertheless contain errors, omissions, or material that is out of date at the time you read it. Neither the authors nor the publisher has any legal responsibility or liability for errors, omissions, out-of-date material, or the reader's application of the medical information or advice contained in this book.

Published on the foundation established in memory of William Chauncey Williams of the Class of 1822, Yale Medical School, and of William Cook Williams of the Class of 1850, Yale Medical School.

Copyright © 2011 by Madhuri Reddy, M.D., M.Sc.
Illustrations copyright © 2011 by Victoria Cansino.

All rights reserved.

This book may not be reproduced, in whole or in part, including illustrations, in any form (beyond that copying permitted by Sections 107 and 108 of the U.S. Copyright Law and except by reviewers for the public press), without written permission from the publishers.

Yale University Press books may be purchased in quantity for educational, business, or promotional use. For information, please e-mail sales.press@yale
.edu (U.S. office) or sales@yaleup.co.uk (U.K. office).

Set in Bulmer type by Newgen North America. Printed in the United States of America.

Library of Congress Cataloging-in-Publication Data

Reddy, Madhuri.
    Healing wounds, healthy skin : a practical guide for patients with chronic wounds / Madhuri Reddy, Rebecca Cottrill ; illustrations by Victoria Cansino.
        p. cm. — (Yale University Press health & wellness)
    Includes bibliographical references and index.
    ISBN 978-0-300-14036-1 (hardback) — ISBN 978-0-300-17100-6 (pbk.)
    1. Wound healing.   2. Wounds and injuries—Treatment.   3. Skin—Care and hygiene.
I. Cottrill, Rebecca.   II. Title.
    RD94.R43 2011
    617.1′06—dc22

                                                                    2011006744

A catalogue record for this book is available from the British Library.
This paper meets the requirements of ANSI/NISO Z39.48-1992 (Permanence of Paper).

10 9 8 7 6 5 4 3 2 1

To all the people who suffer with chronic wounds,
who inspire and teach us

Contents

Acknowledgments

Special thanks to R. Gary Sibbald, M.D.; Elizabeth Ayello, Ph.D., R.N.; Diane Krasner, Ph.D., R.N.; Linda Konner; Jean Thomson Black; Kristin Casady; Foy White-Chu, M.D.; the wound team at the Wound Healing Clinic, The New Women's College Hospital, Toronto, Ontario; and the wound team at Hebrew Rehabilitation Center, Boston, Massachusetts.

Healing Your Wound:
The Top Ten Myths Dispelled

These are what we consider the top ten myths, or common misconceptions, about what can best heal your wounds. Acting on these misbeliefs can make your wounds worse.

1. Myth: Soaking your feet helps a wound heal faster.

TRUTH: Soaking your feet can waterlog the wound and the skin around the wound. This makes the skin more fragile, and puts you at increased risk for microorganisms entering your body and causing a deep infection. The best way to clean your wound is to lightly pat or wipe the wound and surrounding skin with a gentle wound cleanser (such as sterile water or normal saline) that your wound team suggests.

2. Myth: Leaving the wound open to air helps it heal faster.

TRUTH: Leaving the wound open to air can do two harmful things: (1) increase your risk of developing an infection in the wound, and (2) dry out the wound, which makes it less likely to heal. It is best to use a wound dressing to cover the wound at all times (except when you are cleaning it).

3. Myth: Seawater is good for open wounds.

TRUTH: There are a couple of problems with exposing an open wound to seawater. First, the water is not sterile (meaning that it is full of microorganisms that can infect your wound). Second, immersing a wound in any body of water has a similar effect to soaking your feet (see #1, above) and can increase your risk of infection and wound worsening.

4. Myth: Compression bandaging and stockings cut off your circulation.

TRUTH: If your wound team has recommended compression bandaging or stockings, they should first check to ensure that you have good circulation. This may be done with a physical examination or may require specialized testing. Compression needs to be snug to reduce any leg edema (swelling), to help heal your leg wounds, and to prevent future wounds. As long as your wound team has checked to ensure you have adequate circulation and the compression is not unbearably painful or causing your toes to turn bluish, it is not cutting off your circulation.

5. Myth: When your wound team debrides your wound, they are opening it up and making it larger.

TRUTH: Often, your wound may need to be debrided (that is, the dead tissue removed) by your wound team to keep it clean and free of dead tissue, which makes the wound more prone to infection. Sometimes, the wound will appear to be larger after it has been debrided, but this is misleading. Dead tissue hampers healing, even though it can make the wound look like it is healing. Once the dead tissue is removed, the healthy wound underneath is revealed.

6. Myth: When a scab forms, the wound has healed.

TRUTH: This is related to #5, above. Often, a scab is just some dead tissue on top of a wound that can encourage bacteria to grow underneath. Your wound team may decide to debride (that is, remove) this scab, to allow the wound underneath to stay clean.

7. Myth: The best way to heal your wound is to use something new, unusual, or expensive.

TRUTH: The best way to heal a wound is often the simplest way and needs to address the underlying cause of the wound (for example, reduce pressure for bedsores, or wear appropriate shoes for foot ulcers in diabetes). Many unusual therapies do not have good science behind them, may actually make your wound worse, and may be very costly.

8. Myth: Changing the wound dressing every day is better for healing.

TRUTH: Removing the dressing of a chronic wound too frequently can remove new, fragile skin cells that are trying to form, and so may actually impair wound healing. Changing the dressing frequently can also be painful. Most newer wound dressings are meant to be changed every two or three days.

9. Myth: Leg swelling means you have poor circulation.

TRUTH: Although poor circulation may be one cause of leg swelling, there are many other possible causes. It is important to see your wound team and figure out the exact reason your legs are swelling so that you can start to treat the underlying problem.

10. Myth: Loose shoes or slippers don't apply pressure and are good for people with foot wounds.

TRUTH: If you have neuropathy (from diabetes or other causes), loose shoes and slippers can feel comfortable, but can cause friction (rubbing) against the skin, and can actually increase your risk of developing foot wounds. Because of your neuropathy, you cannot feel your feet in your shoes well, so even though shoes may seem comfortable, they may not be protecting your feet from developing wounds. Loose shoes and slippers may not be providing adequate pressure relief in the right places, even if they feel good to you. Therefore, it is important to see a qualified orthotist or podiatrist to ensure that your shoes not only feel good, but are also a perfect fit for your feet.

Preface

What I do is based on powers we all have inside us; the ability to en-dure; the ability to love, to carry on, to make the best of what we have—and you don't have to be a "Superman" to do it.

—CHRISTOPHER REEVE

You have just stubbed your toe. When this used to happen, you would forget about it and it would soon heal. But this time it is differ-ent. This time, here you are several weeks later with a gaping wound in your foot and a raging infection. How did this happen? How will it get better? What is wrong with you?

You have developed what is called a *chronic wound**.

There are many terms used to describe a break in the skin: *wound**, *ulcer**, *sore,* and *bedsore** are a few. These different words all refer to the same thing.

When a break in the skin first occurs, it is known as an "acute" wound. An acute wound most often occurs after a specific traumatic event, such as a burn, surgery, stubbing your toe, or accidentally hit-ting your shin against a shopping cart. Sometimes a wound seems to occur spontaneously and you have no memory of an accident that could explain it.

For a further explanation of words marked with an asterisk (*), see the Glossary of Terms at the back of this book.

In most circumstances, an acute wound heals quickly and easily and does not run into complications like infections. However, when a wound is slow to heal and has not improved within three weeks, it is called a "chronic" wound. A wound can become chronic for many reasons, and caring for these wounds can be complex.

The most common types of chronic wounds include pressure ulcers (also known as bedsores), foot ulcers (most often in people with diabetes), and leg ulcers. Each of these types of chronic wounds, along with more unusual types of wounds, is explained further in later chapters.

Approximately seven million Americans have a slow-to-heal or nonhealing skin wound. This number is likely to grow as the population ages, because older skin does not heal as quickly or as well as younger skin. Pressure ulcers occur in one out of ten people admitted to hospitals, one out of four people in nursing homes, one out of three people with spinal cord injuries, and in 60 percent of spinal cord injury quadriplegics. Chronic wounds can lead to immense pain, suffering, and even death. Pressure ulcers kill 60,000 people per year, which are more deaths than from breast cancer and almost twice as many as from prostate cancer.

One in four people with diabetes will develop a foot wound, which can have very serious consequences. The most common reason that people with diabetes are admitted to the hospital is a foot wound. Persons with diabetes are forty times more likely than persons without diabetes to require an amputation, which is usually the result of infection in a chronic wound and gangrene. More than half of these amputations are preventable. Some 50,000 persons with diabetes per year undergo an amputation; 70 percent of these people will die within five years. Those who undergo a leg amputation also have a 50 percent chance of amputation of the other leg within five years.

This book can help prevent you from being a statistic. While it cannot replace the care and guidance of your health-care providers, it *can* assist you in navigating the sometimes murky waters of finding a good health-care team. This book will also educate you about preventing wounds—in line with the old saying "An ounce of prevention is worth a pound of cure"—as well as review treatment options. It is intended to serve as a valuable, easy-to-use resource guide that contains essential practical information for anyone who has a chronic wound or cares about someone with a chronic wound. Whether you have a chronic wound or you're a caregiver, a friend, or a family member of someone with a chronic wound, *Healing Wounds, Healthy Skin* is a great place to start.

Why Me?

People who develop chronic wounds usually have one or more risk factors that are beyond their control, such as a chronic illness (for example, dementia). You may also have lifestyle factors that put you at even higher risk (for example, smoking). Some people are more likely than others to acquire wounds (for example, people with spinal cord injury), and then be slow to heal or not heal at all (for example, persons with diabetes).

If you are reading this book, you or someone you care about probably falls into one of these categories. Regardless of which category applies, the end result is the same, and you need information about the risks of developing a wound that may become chronic.

Are You at High Risk of Developing a Chronic Wound?

The following questionnaire will help you determine your risk level for a chronic wound.

1. Do you have difficulty walking? (Answer "yes" if you spend some or most of the time in bed, in a chair, or in a wheelchair.)
2. Do you have trouble controlling your bladder and/or bowels?
3. Do you have poor nutrition?
4. Are you very overweight?
5. Do you have diabetes?
7. Do you have poor circulation?
8. Do you have varicose veins?
9. Do you have severe leg swelling?
10. Do you take medications including steroids or others that suppress your immune system for treatment of a disease?

11. Do you have a skin disease?

12. Do you have poor sensation?

If you answered "yes" to *any* of the above questions, you are at risk of developing a wound that may be slow to heal. If you answered "yes" to *more than one* question, you are at even higher risk.

It is important to note that most chronic wounds are *NOT*

- Contagious
- A normal consequence of diabetes
- Inevitable if you live long enough
- Impossible to treat

Difficulties of Having a Chronic Wound

Chronic wounds can be extremely painful, may limit your ability to move, and may make you feel self-conscious especially if they have an odor.

We take for granted that our skin heals: we fall and bruise—it's supposed to heal; we get a cut—it's supposed to close. It can be shocking when seemingly minor injuries not only fail to heal but cause enormous frustration, pain, embarrassment, and financial loss. Perhaps you or a loved one has lost a job because of the time required to care for a chronic wound. What is even more disappointing perhaps is that chronic wounds often initially improve, only to deteriorate because of infection or acute medical illness.

Quality of life is radically altered in people with chronic wounds, because these individuals may spend their limited energy and financial assets searching for answers and seeking out health-care providers skilled enough to treat them. Learning how to live with the physical pain and disability that can come from wounds is a serious challenge. The wound may limit activities, by restricting the ability to walk or swim. Worse than the high financial costs and immense emotional toll are the potentially serious medical consequences of nonhealing chronic wounds: such wounds may sometimes result in sepsis (blood infection), amputation, or even death.

If you have a chronic wound, you are probably already an expert in many aspects of wound care, particularly regarding dressing changes. You have probably experienced the immense frustration of not healing. People with any type of chronic medical problem struggle to find the best health-care providers, the best treatment, and the best way to make life easier and pain-free. Chronic diseases profoundly change the lives of those affected as well as those who love them and may help to take care of them. Whether you are the one with the chronic wound or whether someone you care about has one, this book will help you understand the difficult emotional and physical challenges, and provide you with an abundance of practical information.

How to Use This Book

The best way to get the information you need from this book is to flip to the chapter or chapters that apply to you, to your loved one, or to the particular wound you would like to know more about. Within each chapter, the Healing Hand icon 🖐 will point out important facts to remember, or suggest some handy tips to help you in the prevention or care of your wound. In each chapter we tell the story of a patient that we see or have seen in our clinic, to give you an idea of how other people with chronic wounds manage and to show you that you are not alone (we do not use their real names, of course).

All words or phrases in this book that are followed by an asterisk (*) are explained further in the Glossary of Terms. Every person and every wound is different, and the recommendations and suggestions in this book are only general guidelines. Make sure to talk to your health-care team to determine the specific recommendations that are right for you.

Hope: The Healing Light to Follow

Chronic wounds are serious conditions, but it is not all doom and gloom. Many types of chronic wounds are preventable, with the right information. Most are also treatable with proper care. For example, if diabetic foot ulcers are diagnosed quickly and receive treatment early this may prevent up to 85 percent of amputations.

There is usually a plan that can be put in place to heal these wounds. Often the steps are quite simple. Fortunately, there is increasing evidence regarding the prevention and treatment of chronic wounds, and more health-care professionals are being trained in this field. A multitude of wound care clinics are popping up across the country. And for those wounds that are still not healable, we can improve quality of life and reduce pain. Healable and nonhealable wounds must be managed very differently . . . and we have to have the wisdom—and the information—to be able to know the difference.

One of the best things that people at risk for any of these wounds can do is educate themselves or have a caregiver willing to do the same. Reading this book is the first step in learning more. After reading *Healing Wounds, Healthy Skin,* you will be much more capable of asking your doctor and the rest of your health-care team the right questions, which makes you an effective manager of your own treatment. This book will give you what you need to know in order to make educated choices and decisions that will benefit you. There are many resources out there to help you. You don't have to do it alone.

We applaud your choice to be your own or your loved one's best advocate by learning the causes and treatments of the chronic wounds that affect your life. You are taking steps to heal not only your broken skin but also the broken heart that these wounds have created.

PART ONE

When You Have a Wound That Won't Heal

The skin is the largest organ in the body and is composed of an outer layer and an inner layer. A layer of fatty tissue lies beneath these two layers (Figure 1).

The thickest skin is located on the palms of the hands and on the soles of the feet, and it can be ten times thicker than the thinnest skin, which is found around the eyes and over the eardrums.

What Is Skin?

Skin acts as a protective shield between your vital organs (such as your heart and lungs) and the external world. The skin also acts as a barrier against bacteria and other types of infections. Additionally, skin protects your blood vessels and bones from mechanical injury. For example, when you walk, the soles of the feet withstand a tremendous amount of force, yet the vessels and bones are unharmed.

The top layer of the skin produces the brown pigment melanin*, which gives skin and hair their different colors. The more melanin produced, the darker the skin. Sun exposure stimulates the production of melanin, so your skin becomes darker after you lie out in the sunlight. For more information on how skin pigment can affect wound treatment and healing, see Chapter 25.

The bottom layer of the skin contains an extensive network of small blood vessels. Every square inch of skin contains more than fifteen inches of blood vessels. This inner layer also contains fibers that

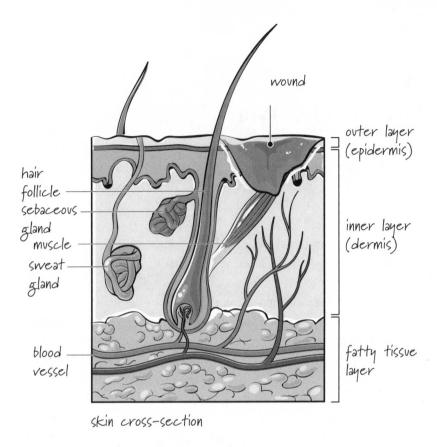

skin cross-section

Figure 1: A cross-section of skin.

contribute to the skin's strength and elasticity (that is, the ability of the skin to bounce back to its original shape after it has been stretched). It also contains lymphatic vessels, which help to remove waste products. When lymphatic vessels are damaged or blocked, it can result in severe swelling and lymphedema*. For more information on lymphedema, see Chapter 12.

The inner layer of the skin also contains nerve fibers, which is why wounds which are not that deep (that is, just go to the inner layer of skin) or are healing can sometimes be more painful than wounds that are much deeper. Nerve endings in the skin allow you to take in sensory information from the world around you. They help you to avoid injury by making you aware of pain, pressure, heat, and cold. Sensation allows us to identify potential dangers and avoid injury.

If you lose your sense of touch (this happens in some people with diabetes, especially on the soles of their feet), your risk of injury increases. Wounds can then result, and you may not even know it until they become severe or infected (see Chapter 8). Anything that impairs the ability to sense pressure, including the use of pain medications or sleeping pills, spinal cord lesions, or cognitive impairment, puts the patient at risk for trauma. If you—or the person you care for—can't feel the growing discomfort of pressure and respond to it, you cannot protect yourself from injury.

An important function of the skin is its role in your appearance. The skin is the largest organ in the body and the most visible, and as a result can have an enormous impact on your self-esteem and social acceptance (ask any teenager with acne!). A wound can severely undermine the way you feel about yourself, and other people may find it difficult to accept those whose skin is not "normal." These emotional and practical considerations are important and should be addressed as part of the healing process, in addition to the medical issues.

1
How Wounds Heal

Any break in the skin is considered a wound*. The severity of a wound depends on how much damage there is: a wound can vary from a superficial break in the top layer of skin to deep trauma that involves the muscle and bone.

Healing a wound is like rebuilding a damaged house (Figure 2). The construction of a house is made up of a series of organized and synchronized processes. Without the right signals at the right time, a house cannot be rebuilt, nor will a wound be healed. Think of blood flow to the wound as the workers that build the house. Think of the nutrition as the materials used to build the house. If the workers (the blood flow) and the materials (the nutrition) are not present in the correct amount, the house (that is, the healing wound) will be weak and incomplete.

A wound destroys the skin and underlying tissues just as a hurricane destroys a house and its foundation. Arteries, veins, and nerves become exposed just as plumbing and electrical wires are exposed. The initial phases of construction are to cap these wires in order to prevent further destruction and loss. Capping the wires is like the clotting phase of wound healing. The clotting phase is where blood flow from the wound is stopped. The body sends chemicals to the wound that thicken the blood and plug the flow of blood. Next, just as skilled workers begin their expert work, specialized cells begin to reinforce the wound and erect outside barriers. These barriers protect the weak, compromised interior. Over the next several months, wound remodeling occurs in order to reduce the size of the scar while increasing the scar's strength and protective quality.

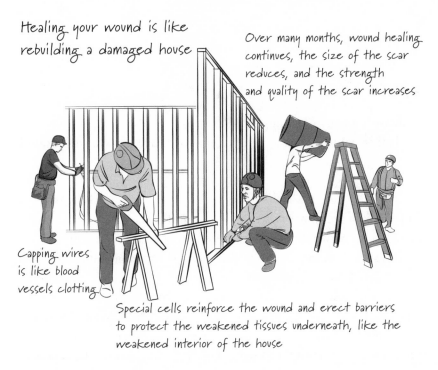

Healing your wound is like rebuilding a damaged house

Over many months, wound healing continues, the size of the scar reduces, and the strength and quality of the scar increases

Capping wires is like blood vessels clotting

Special cells reinforce the wound and erect barriers to protect the weakened tissues underneath, like the weakened interior of the house

If, at any time, this process gets "stuck" (that is, wound healing is interrupted), healing is slowed and a chronic wound results.

Figure 2: Healing a wound is like rebuilding a damaged house.

At any time, the proper order of the phases of wound healing may be interrupted. When this occurs, the healing process gets "stuck" and does not follow the sequence it is supposed to. This results in what is called a chronic (or nonhealing) wound*. Certain conditions, such as diabetes and autoimmune diseases (for example, multiple sclerosis), and certain medications (for example, steroids and some anti-inflammatory medications) may delay wound healing.

A house requires a foundation and framing structure, with basic key materials. Similarly, wound healing is slow when the building materials of adequate health, nutrition (such as protein, carbohydrates, fat, fluids, vitamins, and minerals), oxygen (which is available if there is good blood flow), and a well-functioning immune system are lacking. When the skin is injured, its normal barrier function is broken. Typically, inflammation begins in order to protect the internal organs. If you have a strong immune system, superficial injuries heal spontaneously without any complications.

If this natural healing progression is delayed, a chronic wound may result.

The Different Ways That Wounds Heal

Wounds can heal in one of two ways.

A superficial acute wound (for example, a first-degree burn) or a surgical cut usually heals when the skin's outer layer (the epithelium) closes by growing in from the edges of the wound and out from skin cells lining the hair follicles and sweat glands. These wounds usually heal in four to fourteen days.

Once this time period has passed, and if the wound is not showing any signs of healing, it becomes too late to heal in this way, and the wound then has to heal another way: from the inside out. Deep wounds with edges that are unable to easily be lined up together also heal in this way. They fill up on the inside with tissue first, then a scar forms and, finally, the skin's outer layer grows closed, mostly from the wound edges. Chronic wounds (such as pressure ulcers, burns, surgical wounds that do not heal right away, and traumatic injuries) heal in this way. These wounds take longer to heal, result in scarring, and have a higher rate of complications (such as infection). This is why it is not possible to simply put stitches in a chronic wound: you are still left with a hole underneath the sutured area. This is why chronic wounds need to be healed from the bottom up (that is, from the inside out).

Factors That Affect Healing

The healing process is affected by many factors. We discuss many of these in more detail in later chapters in the book.

- *Nutrition.* Nutrition is one of the most important factors in wound healing. Malnutrition is a common finding in people with chronic wounds (see Chapter 32).
- *Oxygen.* Wound healing requires a regular supply of oxygen. For example, oxygen is critical for white blood cells to destroy bacteria. If the supply is hindered by poor blood flow to the area of the wound, healing will be slowed. Possible causes of inadequate blood flow to the area of the wound include pressure or vascular disease (see Part IV).
- *Infection.* Infection may occur in the wound only, or spread into the blood and rest of the body. Any break in the skin allows bacteria to enter the wound. Any wound that occurs outside of the sterile surgical environment contains bacteria, which are important to the healthy functioning of skin. Just because bacteria are present in the wound does not mean they have invaded and caused infection. An infection occurs when bacteria overwhelm the wound and cause damage to the wound. Some signs of infection are new or increased pain, redness, heat, and drainage. Healing cannot progress until the infection is treated (see Chapter 15).
- *Age.* Healing in older adults is slower but ultimately is as effective as that of younger adults (see Chapter 23).
- *Chronic health conditions.* Respiratory problems, poor circulation, diabetes, and cancer can increase the risk of wounds and interfere with wound healing. These conditions can interfere with proper oxygen supply to the wound and also with nutrition, both of which affect healing. Many of these health conditions will be reviewed in detail in several other chapters throughout this book.
- *Medications.* Any medications that reduce movement or level of consciousness (such as sleeping pills, sedatives, and tranquilizers) have the potential to inhibit the ability to sense and respond to pressure. Furthermore, because movement promotes adequate blood flow and therefore oxygen to the skin, lack of motion means that blood near the skin delivers less oxygen than it should.

Some medications, such as steroids and chemotherapy, weaken the body's ability to heal properly. This can be a big problem, especially in those with impaired immune systems.

- *Smoking.* Carbon monoxide, a component of cigarette smoke, replaces oxygen in the blood. This reduces the amount of oxygen in the bloodstream, resulting in a decreased ability for the body to heal a wound. This also occurs in people regularly exposed to secondhand smoke.

- *Being overweight.* Being significantly overweight can interfere with wound healing. There may be reduced oxygen near the wound, increased tension in the skin around the wound, skin folds that may keep the wound moist and allow bacteria to accumulate, or there may also be associated medical conditions (such as diabetes) that reduce the ability to heal.

In addition, someone who is overweight may actually be malnourished and so may be lacking the essential minerals and vitamins necessary for proper wound healing (see Chapter 26).

2

Recognizing Your Fears

When your wound persists, you and your loved one may experience a variety of emotions ranging from anger, denial, and anxiety to depression. These feelings don't occur in any particular order and vary from person to person. You may also experience emotions that are not directly related to the slowly healing wound, such as fear of what the future holds and worries about work or finances.

Before you can take any positive steps towards feeling better, it's important to identify your fears. In this chapter, we will address some of the more common fears associated with a prolonged nonhealing wound, starting with those most frequently experienced by the person with the wound, followed by an overview of common caregivers'

In coping with a severe chronic wound, one of the biggest fears and frustrations for both the person with the wound and family is the unknown. No one can predict how the wound will progress for you or foresee how it will affect you and those you love. Only one thing is certain: it is possible to improve quality of life for everyone involved.

fears. Sometimes you and your caregiver may share many of the same fears. We hope that by discussing these issues, you will realize that you are not alone, trying to solve unheard-of, irresolvable problems. Some suggestions for coping and management are included along the way.

Remember that you're not alone and that any fears you have are natural and common in people with chronic wounds.

Common Fears of the Person with the Wound

Whether your nonhealing wound is relatively recent or you have had it for a while, or if you care for someone with a nonhealing wound, you may find that some of the concerns we discuss here are familiar to you. This section is intended to help you understand your own fears and how these fears may be affecting you, affecting your ability to heal, and affecting your quality of life. Here are some experiences of people with nonhealing wounds struggling through difficult situations:

- I have diabetes and a wound on my foot that won't go away. I always worried that I would have to have an *amputation*, and this is the first sign. There is no point in me taking care of this wound, since an amputation with diabetes is inevitable.
- My loved one, who has Alzheimer's disease and is mostly bed bound, has developed a bedsore. Bedsores are a *sign of the end of life*. This is the beginning of the end, and there is nothing left for me to do except mourn the inevitable loss of my spouse.
- I have leg ulcers that have a terrible smell. Everyone, from my coworkers to people in the grocery line, can smell them. It is repulsive, and I am so *embarrassed*.
- I have a wound on my foot, and it seems to be moving in the right direction toward healing, and it doesn't even hurt . . . but there are no guarantees, right? Just because it seems OK right now doesn't mean that it couldn't deteriorate at any time. I am so *scared of developing an infection or something worse* at any time.

- I have Parkinson's disease and get around mostly with a wheelchair. I have a new sore on my backside that is *unbelievably painful*. It keeps me from enjoying life, even the time I have with my grandchildren. But a sore from a wheelchair is inevitable, and pain with age and my condition is a fact of life. It scares me that the pain is going to continue, get worse, and keep making my life miserable.
- All these dressings are so *expensive*, and my insurance will not cover them. Apparently there are techniques that could really help me heal, but they cost thousands of dollars. Plus, my health-care team tells me I should stay off work for a while until I heal, but I'm self-employed and have no unemployment insurance. How am I supposed to feed myself? How do I support my family?
- The nurses showed me how to do the dressing. But how do I know whether I am doing it correctly? It frightens and worries me that I am not applying the dressing exactly as they instructed me to. What if I'm missing signs of infection? How do I know when the wound is worse? I am trying my best but perhaps this wound isn't healing because *I'm doing something wrong*.
- I had a spinal cord injury and am in a wheelchair. Now I have a pressure sore. I'm a young man, married with small children. As if my being in a wheelchair wasn't enough inconvenience, my wife now has to do the dressings on my wound. I worry about being a *burden* on her.

How to Address Specific Fears and Worries

Having a wound that is slow to heal can cause people to react in many different ways. No two people respond in exactly the same way. Finding out the cause of the wound allows you to educate yourself about the condition and seek appropriate treatment, thereby avoiding unnecessary treatments or workups.

You can take a more active role in your own treatment by becoming aware of the specific cause or causes of the wound. The earlier you seek help for the wound, the more likely the wound is to heal, and not develop complications such as infections. You should also discuss any fears you may have about living with a chronic (and sometimes progressive) medical condition with your health-care practitioner.

AMPUTATION

If you have a leg or foot ulcer, fear of amputation is very common. Talk to your health-care team. If your health-care team feels you need an amputation but you would like to get another opinion, get a second opinion. It is your right.

An amputation requires other complicating factors in addition to the leg or foot wound. Amputations are usually done because of a non-healing foot or leg wound in individuals who also have terrible circulation, a very high risk of infection, and/or uncontrollable pain.

Sometimes, people who have had a prolonged nonhealing wound for years and have tried many treatments and complications come to feel that an amputation may actually improve their quality of life. There are people who are happier after their amputation than they were before.

A SIGN OF DYING

In someone with advanced dementia, a bedsore (or pressure ulcer) may be a sign that the person is near the end of their life. Pressure ulcers may not be preventable in this situation (for more information, see Part II). Maintaining quality of life then becomes the primary issue (see Chapter 31).

EMBARRASSMENT

The odor of a wound is usually more obvious to the person with the wound than it is to others. There are steps that can be taken to address and reduce odors (see Chapter 31).

INFECTION

No one can tell if or when a wound will suddenly get infected and worsen, but there are things you can do to drastically reduce the risk of your wound getting infected (see Chapter 15).

PAIN

Your health-care team should work to help alleviate your pain. Your quality of life is important, and undertreated pain is a serious medical concern (see Chapter 34).

FINANCIAL CONSEQUENCES

Managing wounds can be very expensive, not just in terms of costs of treatment, but also in terms of time off work. Discuss your concerns with your health-care provider and wound care team. Options are available in terms of less expensive dressings and return to work with limited responsibilities. Your wound care team will not know that these areas concern you unless you talk with them about it (see Chapter 39).

BEING A BURDEN TO LOVED ONES

Sometimes, a person with a nonhealing wound fears becoming a burden to his or her loved one because he or she depends on a family member to change dressings or otherwise assist with care.

There are strategies that can help you preserve your self-reliance. Your health-care team can answer any specific questions you may have about your own situation.

Common Concerns of the Caregiver

If you're responsible for caring for a loved one with a nonhealing wound, your concerns may be:

- Fear that you are not managing the wound properly
- Worry about finances
- Responsibilities as the primary caregiver
- Worry about your loved one and fearing the loss of them
- Worry about yourself and your family

We will address many of these issues in many later chapters, and focus even more on the caregiver in Chapter 37.

Take-Home Message

It is important to discuss any fears you have with your health-care team. Don't assume that they can read your mind, and don't be embarrassed by what is bothering you. Remember, most fears discussed in this chapter are actually pretty common in people with chronic wounds. If you feel that your worries are not being heard and addressed, get a second opinion from another wound care specialist.

3
Creating Your Health-Care Team
It Takes a Village

The health-care system can be a complex maze that is difficult to navigate. Having to visit several different health-care specialists (as many people with chronic wounds do) can aggravate this already confusing situation. To help you avoid as many health-care challenges as possible, we will show you how to find and coordinate the care and support you need. It helps enormously to be well informed about your medical issues and your own care. We'll assist you with strategies to achieve this goal, and also will help you understand some of the language that your wound team may use.

The number of health-care professionals who have the expertise and experience to help you manage your wound is available and growing. Unfortunately, it can be challenging to separate the good wound care providers from the not-as-good ones. We'll show you how to scout out the best.

Who's Who on Your Wound Care Team

Many different types of health-care professionals are well trained at managing your chronic wound. Any wound clinic you decide to work with should be interdisciplinary, i.e., have more than one type of health-care professional working to care for your wound. These health-care professionals may all be in the same wound center, or may work in different centers. Usually, one main wound care center coordinates your care by identifying your treatment needs and referring you to the specialists who can best address them.

The key thing to know is that *you* are the most important person on your health-care team.

Depending on the type of wound you have and what type of underlying medical issues are affecting you and your wound's healing process, your wound care team should consist of at least two or more of the following specialists:

> Dietician*
> Doctor
> Nurse
> Physiotherapist*/Occupational therapist*
> Podiatrist*/Chiropodist*
> Social worker*

You may have more than one doctor on your team. Your doctor may be a primary care physician training in wound care and/or may be one of these specialists:

> Dermatologist*
> Endocrinologist*
> Geriatrician*
> Infectious diseases specialist
> Orthopedic surgeon*
> Physical medicine and rehabilitation specialist*
> Plastic surgeon*
> Psychiatrist*
> Vascular surgeon*

Not all physicians are trained in the management of chronic wounds. You should find out what the doctor's training and experience in the area are, and determine if he or she has had any additional training in wound care. For some doctors, this may be Certified Wound Specialist (CWS) or other certification, for some it is a fellowship (that is, extra training after medical school and residency), and for others it may be some courses and conferences in addition to experience. You might feel awkward asking your doctor about his or her training or credentials, but it is your right as a patient to do so. Remember, your best chances for managing your wound improve by acting as your own strongest advocate.

If you don't live near a wound specialist, you may be able to see the specialist intermittently and your local health-care team more frequently. The specialist can provide recommendations for your own team to follow. You may need to travel or pay to go to a specialist, but the peace of mind you get knowing that you're receiving the best care and guidance possible is well worth it.

Finding the Right Team for You

Depending on the type of chronic wound you have, your relationship with your wound specialist may be a long and personal one. You may at times discuss very private topics such as leaky bladder or uncontrollable bowels. It's important to find someone you feel comfortable with. Some key elements of successful relationships are trust, good communication, and mutual respect.

Accessibility of the Wound Center

Find out how accessible the wound center is. Even if you aren't having any mobility problems at the moment, you never know when you may need good accessibility. It is amazing how many wound centers and doctors' offices are not accessible to people with canes or walkers or in wheelchairs and on stretchers. You need a wound center that is easy to get to, so check out the accessibility ahead of time. A phone call to the office will do: ask about proximity of parking, whether there are stairs or an elevator, and so on. Nothing is more frustrating than making your way to a doctor's office only to find that you have to park several blocks away or climb a flight of stairs.

A Team Player

The best wound specialists know that chronic wound care involves a lot of teamwork. They recognize the invaluable contributions made by all health-care professionals. Your wound specialist needs to work collaboratively with other specialists and team members in order to provide you the most effective care. The specialist who feels that he or she is the only provider you need is probably not your best bet.

Bedside Manner

You need to decide what personality qualities are most important to you in a wound care specialist. You may want someone you feel is pleasant and courteous above all else, or you may want expertise most of all. You may find all these qualities in the same person, but not everyone is so fortunate. You need to find someone you trust and feel comfortable with.

Communication

Find out whether the nurse or other health-care professional at the wound center is available for phone calls. Most wound clinics don't take calls during the day, but you should be able to leave a message and get a return call from the doctor or nurse within a reasonable period of time (within two to four days is reasonable). Having this kind of communication with the wound center is important because questions about dressings and wound worsening are common. You'll find it comforting to know that you can count on getting a call back when you have a question or concern. Of course, in the case where you need to see a doctor right away, you'll need to call either your primary care doctor or visit the nearest emergency room.

Ability to Face Things Head-On

A chronic wound can interfere with your life and lifestyle. You will need to be able to talk with your wound specialist about treatment and quality of life decisions you're trying to make with the expectation that he or she will answer honestly and thoughtfully. If your doctor doesn't seem willing or comfortable having these kinds of conversations with you, it's probably time to look for another doctor.

It is important to have a wound specialist who doesn't avoid difficult topics. Some wound specialists may give false assurances and tell you the wound is healing when it may not be. If you have a wound that may never heal, you need a specialist who tells you that, so you can plan with that knowledge (also see Chapter 31). Therefore look for a specialist you can trust to be forthright and realistic with you about your chronic wound.

How to Make the Most of Your Health-Care Appointments

As the most important member of your health-care team, you have responsibilities that will help you get the best care possible. Often, your treatment is only as good as the information you provide. Here are some tips:

- *Bring a list.* Bring a list of your medications, names and numbers of all the doctors—and wound specialists if applicable—you are currently seeing (or have seen over the past few years), and any letters or blood work results from your health-care providers.

  Make sure to keep your wound team informed about any new medications (over-the-counter and prescription) and treatments that you're using for any of your medical issues. In fact, keeping a complete list in your wallet for easy reference is a good idea. It's important to keep your wound team informed because over-the-counter products may contain ingredients that may interact with drugs or treatments that your team may prescribe for you.
- *Be prepared.* It's a good idea to prepare a list of questions ahead of time, write them down, and make sure the most important ones are at the top of the list. This way you won't forget to ask something you need to know during your visit. If

you run out of time during the visit, you'll have had a chance to ask the most important ones.

- *Don't hold back.* Speak up when you're concerned. The wound specialist can't read your mind, so don't hesitate to talk about your symptoms and concerns.
- *Bring an extra pair of ears.* Most people aren't at their most relaxed state when they are in a doctor's office. Or, you may have some memory issues that make it difficult to remember what the wound specialist says. To head off any forgetfulness or worry, you may want to bring a relative or friend along to listen. It's also okay to ask your specialist to write down the key points, particularly relating to the diagnosis and treatment.
- *Be on time.* Everyone gets frustrated when forced to wait in a doctor's office, but sometime, people arriving late is one reason that doctors fall behind. Often, the doctor is trying to give each patient the attention he or she needs (which may not always be predictable ahead of time), and some people with complex medical problems take longer than others. One day it may be your appointment that runs over the scheduled time.

Getting a Second Opinion

Nearly one in three adults in the United States never seek a second opinion for their diagnosis, and nearly one in ten never fully understand their diagnosis. But chronic wound care is a combination of art and science, and there are many questions with no single right answer. Therefore, specialists have different opinions on how to handle many aspects of chronic wound care.

1. Getting a second opinion allows you not only to confirm the diagnosis, but also to get a different perspective on your treatment options. Some wound specialists are more conservative and others more aggressive. There may be good arguments for several different options. By getting a second opinion, you get to hear *all* of your options.

2. It is also possible that another specialist might come up with a completely different and more promising option—one that your first specialist didn't think of, or didn't know about. No doctor can know everything or make the right decision all the time.

3. A second opinion can also serve as a quality check—to make sure you're really getting the most current and most effective treatment.

4. Second opinions are particularly valuable if your wound is not healing and your specialist recommends undesirable treatments (for example, an amputation) or potentially expensive treatments (just because it's expensive doesn't mean it's going to work). You should investigate as you would for any big financial commitment. Any time you're considering a procedure that has a risk of death, stroke, or severe infection, you should also get a second opinion.

Whom Do I Ask for a Second Opinion?

There are several ways to go about getting a second opinion. The steps for getting a second opinion appear in Figure 3.

Ask your wound specialist for a recommendation. Ask for the name of another doctor or specialist, so you can get a second opinion. Don't worry about hurting your specialist's feelings. Most doctors welcome a second opinion, especially when surgery or long-term treatment is involved. In fact, if your doctor gets upset or angry about your wanting to seek a second opinion . . . it's time to find another doctor.

Ask someone you trust for a recommendation. If you don't feel comfortable asking your doctor for a referral, then call another doctor you trust. You can also call university teaching hospitals and medical societies in your area for the names of doctors. Some of this information is also available on the Internet.

Check with your health insurance provider. Call your insurance company before you get a second opinion. Ask if they will pay

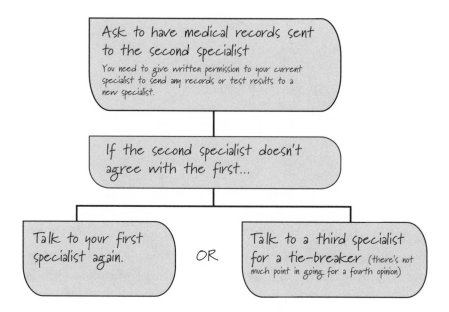

Ask to have medical records sent to the second specialist
You need to give written permission to your current specialist to send any records or test results to a new specialist.

If the second specialist doesn't agree with the first...

Talk to your first specialist again.

OR

Talk to a third specialist for a tie-breaker (there's not much point in going for a fourth opinion)

Figure 3: Getting a second opinion. Should you ask for one?

for this office visit. Many health insurance providers do. Ask if there are any special procedures you or your primary care doctor need to follow.

Once you get an opinion you trust and make a decision on your course of treatment, it is best that you stick with that provider rather than switching back and forth or going to see more than one provider at a time. This ensures that you get the best, most streamlined care possible.

If It Gets to Be Too Overwhelming

If at any point the decisions and information start to feel unmanageable, you may be able to access a care manager. Care managers are professionals who are trained to help coordinate your care and identify helpful community resources. Your primary care doctor or your wound team will likely be able to refer you to a care manager.

4
Your Initial Visit with the Wound Team

Finding out what caused your wound in the first place is the most important part in healing it. This investigation may involve one or more medical tests. In this chapter, we describe the various tests your wound care team may have to do to make a diagnosis and find the cause for any other symptoms you may be having.

One of the factors that may complicate this process is that there is not always one specific test or type of X-ray that can be used to find the wound's cause. Finding the cause of chronic wounds requires some detective work. This may include the need for your wound care team to piece together information from a variety of sources, including your medical history, the symptoms you report, the results of the physical examination, and other tests that may be performed.

Medical History

The wound team's ability to piece together the evidence (your symptoms, physical changes, etc.) and figure out the cause of the wound is only as good as the information that the team is given. Come to the appointment with all your medical records and test results. Be prepared to answer questions about past and present complaints, relevant family history, activities of daily living (what you are able to do for yourself: bathing, shopping, etc.), and any medications you take. This information is valuable in three ways:

- It helps the wound team rule out other problems (for example, if you don't have diabetes, other causes for your wound can be considered).
- It lets the wound team know whether you have any family history relevant to the wound (for example, varicose veins can be hereditary and result in leg wounds).
- It can indicate whether inability to perform activities of daily living, or immobility, is a cause of your wounds (such as pressure sores from lying in bed too long).

While taking your medical history, the wound specialist will evaluate your symptoms, which are the problems or changes you're reporting. Because every person experiences and describes symptoms differently, they are subjective—that is, based on your feelings and thoughts. However, just because symptoms are subjective doesn't make your symptoms less important, it just means that the specialist has to rely on your experience of them to try to get a handle on what the problems may be and how severe they are (Figure 4).

Bringing a family member, caregiver, loved one, or friend along to the appointment with your wound team is always a good idea. Other people in your life may be able to offer some insights to your team that you didn't think of, and may also help you to remember what the health-care professionals said to you.

The point is, don't show up empty-handed for your appointment with the wound care team. You are the most important person on your wound care team. You play an essential role in making sure you receive an accurate diagnosis and effective treatment of your wound.

Physical Exam

The physical exam is an important tool for diagnosing the cause of your wound and for determining whether or not there is an infection in the wound. As part of the physical exam, the specialist will also be looking for evidence of things that you may have never even noticed.

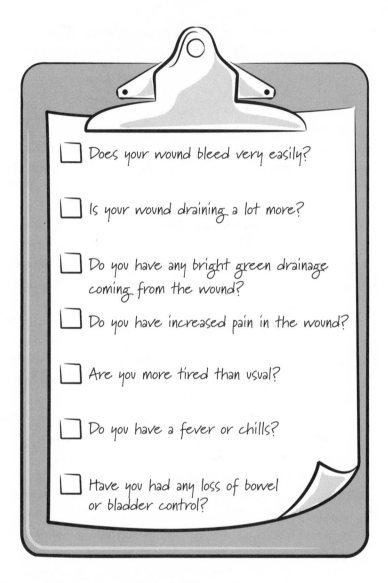

Figure 4: What your wound specialist may ask you.

The physical exam that your medical team does will evaluate one or more of the following:

- *The wound itself.* By looking at the wound itself, the specialist may be able to determine its cause and to start treating it more quickly. The location of the wound is particularly helpful in determining its cause, whether the wound is due to pressure points or to poor circulation, for example. The wound specialist will also be looking at the tissue inside the wound to see if it looks healthy, overgrown, or infected. The skin at the edge of the wound (the wound border*) can also be helpful in diagnosing certain types of chronic wounds (such as pyoderma gangrenosum*, discussed further in Chapter 16).
- *The skin surrounding the wound.* The skin around the wound can be as important as the wound itself. Red skin, for example, can sometimes be the first sign of infection. Irritated, itchy skin may also be the result of infection and drainage in the wound, or an allergy from a product you may be using on the wound. Discolored skin is often a sign of venous stasis*, discussed further in Chapter 10. Certain changes in the texture and thickness of the skin are seen in lymphedema* (explained in Chapter 12).
- *The skin on the rest of your body.* For some types of wounds, it is particularly important to examine the rest of the body. For example, if you have a foot wound and you have diabetes, it is important that your wound specialist examines your other foot too, to make sure it is not at risk of developing the same type of wound. If your mobility is decreased, the wound specialist needs to look at all the pressure points on your body to make sure you don't have early signs of pressure sores anywhere else. A wound specialist will look at other areas of skin, not just the part that bothers you the most, in order to help prevent future problems.
- *Swelling in the legs.* Swelling, or edema, can help tell how severe an underlying disease, such as venous stasis, is. Your doctor may press on your legs to see how deep and for how

long an impression is left in the skin. This helps to tell the severity of the edema. Swelling also occurs with blood clots and infection.

- *Pulses in the feet.* If you have a foot wound, your wound specialist will feel for pulses in the feet to help determine whether there is enough blood flow to allow your wound to heal. If the specialist cannot feel any pulses, he or she may order further investigations to see exactly how much blood flow is present (for more information on these investigations, see Chapter 10). This helps the specialist decide on what dressings to use, if compression is appropriate, and whether other treatment would be effective.

- *Sensation in the feet.* An important risk factor for wound development in the feet is the inability to feel normally, also known as reduced sensation (see Chapter 8). This occurs most often in people with diabetes, but poor sensation can occur in people that do not have diabetes as well. One way that your specialist can determine the degree of sensation is by using a monofilament*.

- *Skin temperature.* It is important to determine whether there is infection in the wound. Some ways of telling include increased drainage, increased odor, or increased pain and redness. However, these signs may not always be present, so your specialist may make use of another examination tool, skin temperature. Simply feeling the skin with the specialist's own hand can be helpful but is not always reliable. Use of an infrared thermometer* can be useful and more reliable.

- *Your mobility.* Depending on the location of your wound, the specialist may ask you to walk, shift weight, or move your feet or ankles. For example, if your mobility is poor, you are at increased risk for developing and worsening any pressure sores. If you are unable to move your ankle through its full range of normal motion, this may increase your risk for development or poor healing of a venous ulcer*. If your ability to walk normally is impaired, it may increase your risk for wounds on the feet.

Lab Tests, Imaging, and Other Ways of Taking a Good Look at Your Wound

Your medical history and physical examination alone are not usually enough to show the underlying cause of the wound or diagnose infection. Therefore, your wound specialist is likely to order one or more of the following tests:

- *Swab* (also known as a wound culture). If your wound specialist suspects that there may be an infection in your wound, he or she may do a swab*. He or she will use a cotton-tipped swab (sort of like a Q-tip) and wipe a part of the wound with it, put it into a container, and send it to the lab for analysis. The result from a swab is one tool your specialist uses to diagnose infection.
- *Blood work*. Blood tests can reveal if the white blood cell count (one way your body fights infection) is high. Blood work can also tell the average blood sugar (if you have diabetes) over the last three months.
- *X-rays*. X-rays sometimes show damage to bone from infection.
- *Bone scan*. A bone scan is a nuclear scanning test (don't worry—this is a sound medical investigation and not a way to make you radioactive). The scan identifies new areas of bone growth or breakdown, and can evaluate bone infection. A bone scan can often detect a problem days to months earlier than a regular X-ray test, but for a wound that has been present for a long time, a bone scan is not as good as some other types of tests.
- *MRI*. Magnetic resonance imaging (MRI) scans are a highly sophisticated test and, as such, are very expensive. They can be worth the expense, though: MRIs are one of the best tests to see if there is a bone infection.
- *CT scan*. Computed tomography, commonly known as a CT scan, combines multiple X-ray images with the aid of a computer to produce cross-sectional views of the body. CT scans

can also help to see if there is a bone infection, particularly if
you can't have an MRI for some reason.

- *Biopsy.* A biopsy is a sample of skin or bone that is taken and
  sent to a pathologist, who looks under a microscope to make a
  diagnosis.
  - —Skin biopsy. A skin biopsy is a procedure in which a doctor
    cuts and removes a small sample of skin to have it tested.
    The skin sample is looked at under a microscope for
    cancer, infection, or other disorders. The doctor will first
    cleanse the biopsy site, and then numb the skin by using
    an anesthetic (pain-relieving) spray, cream, or injection. A
    small piece of skin is then cut out using one of a few differ-
    ent techniques. Sometimes stitches are needed to close the
    site, but they may not be needed. The procedure is usually
    done in the doctor's office. When the biopsy is performed
    you may have some soreness around the biopsied site for
    one to two weeks. Tylenol (acetaminophen) is usually suf-
    ficient to relieve any discomfort. If you had stitches after
    the procedure, keep the area as clean and as dry as pos-
    sible. Your doctor will tell you when the stitches should be
    removed (usually within one week). If adhesive steri-strips
    (which look like small pieces of tape) were used to close the
    incision, do not remove them. They will gradually fall off
    on their own. If the strips do not fall off on their own, your
    health-care provider will remove them at your next follow-
    up appointment.
  - —Bone biopsy. A bone biopsy is a procedure in which a small
    sample of bone is taken from the body and looked at under
    a microscope for cancer, infection, or other bone disorders.
    Bone biopsies are done usually to see if there is an infection
    in the bone, especially if there were problems seen on X-ray.
    The sample of bone can be removed by inserting a needle
    through the skin and directly into the bone or by cutting
    through the skin to expose an area of the bone. With either
    type of procedure, anesthetic is provided to prevent pain.

In Case of Emergency:
When to Call Your Wound Specialist

With a chronic wound, your wound specialist may schedule clinic visits anywhere from every four weeks to every eight weeks or more, depending on the type of wound you have. However, if you develop new symptoms or the wound is worsening, it is important to call your wound specialist or your primary care physician right away, since these symptoms could indicate an infection, allergy, or need to change current treatment. If you notice any of the following, call your health-care professional for further instructions:

- There is increased drainage from the wound
- There is green drainage from the wound
- Your ulcer is bleeding (apply pressure for ten minutes and if it is still bleeding, notify your wound team)
- There is significantly increased pain in the wound
- There is new redness around the wound
- You have developed a new wound
- You have developed a rash
- You have developed fever or chills
- You have developed severe diarrhea or vomiting from any antibiotics prescribed to you by your wound specialist
- The wound is getting bigger between clinic visits

However, the latter procedure usually requires general anesthesia.

- *Pressure mapping*: Pressure mapping technology is an evaluation tool that consists of a computer, pressure mapping software, a flexible sensor pad, an electronics unit, and a power source. The pad is positioned under areas susceptible to pressure (such as under your backside), and the results are mapped on a computer. Pressure map images show areas of high and low pressure while seated.

- *Blood flow tests*: Blood flow tests are useful to help to see how good your circulation is, which can affect the healing of your wound. We discuss this further in Chapter 11.

PART TWO

Pressure Sores

Pressure sores are known by many different names: bedsores, decubitus ulcers, or pressure ulcers. Nearly 3 million Americans have one or more pressure sores. Pressure sores are a serious health problem, particularly in certain populations, such as residents of nursing homes, patients in hospitals, older persons, and people with paraplegia.

All tissues in the body (whether skin, muscle, or fat) depend on blood circulation for the oxygen and nutrients they need. Compression of these tissues (from immobility, for example) interferes with circulation, reducing or completely cutting off blood flow. The result, known as ischemia*, is that tissues fail to receive adequate supplies of oxygen and nutrients. Unless the pressure relents, portions of these tissues eventually die. Skin is tougher than some of the deeper tissues, so by the time you see tissue damage in the skin, there is a good chance that damage has already occurred in deeper tissues.

The pressure resulting from a person's decreased mobility occurs because the skin and the tissues underneath the skin are tightly pinched between a surface (such as a mattress or a chair) and a bone. The blood vessels at the skin are quite small and collapse quite easily with relatively little pressure. When you are sick, the blood vessels collapse even more easily. When you are not able to move around well, unrelenting pressure may occur. As a result of this continual pressure over several hours or days, irreversible damage occurs to the skin and underlying tissues.

Pressure sores can increase your risk of infection and even the risk of death. They can also be painful. Preventing them means that you'll

Myth: Pressure sores are an inevitable consequence of old age.
Truth: Pressure sores can often be prevented, no matter how old you are.

be able to prevent other health complications, as well as avoid prolonged and expensive hospitalizations. If you have a serious underlying medical problem, the pressure sore itself may seem to be the least of your concerns, but developing one may cause a serious negative impact on your health and quality of life.

Health professionals, government agencies, and insurers have all started to take preventing pressure sores seriously. Healthy People 2010 (a report of America's health-care goals) includes a goal of halving the frequency of pressure sores in nursing homes. As of October 2008, the Centers for Medicare and Medicaid Services (CMS), the federal insurance program for adults over sixty-five years of age and for the disabled, has stopped paying hospitals for care resulting from large pressure sores that started while someone was admitted to the hospital. CMS hopes to encourage hospitals to do more to prevent these situations of less than optimal care. Insurers often follow CMS's lead. Health-care professionals share your concerns about the seriousness of pressure sores, and your wound care team is there to help you prevent and treat them.

5
Why Do Pressure Sores Happen?

Mrs. E is a healthy eighty-six-year-old retired schoolteacher. Last winter, she slipped on some ice and fractured her hip. She was admitted to the hospital in order to have surgery to repair her hip. After the surgery she was not able to move around for several days, and she developed an area of redness on her lower back. This area of redness went on to become a pressure sore.

Mr. H, a patient in our clinic, has had quadriplegia (that is, paralysis from the neck down) for fifty years. He was doing well until recently, when he changed to a new lift that assisted him in getting out of bed and into his wheelchair. This lift placed pressure on the same area each time it was used, causing friction and rubbing on a daily basis, eventually resulting in a pressure sore.

What Exactly Causes a Pressure Sore?

If you have difficulty moving around, such as after a spinal cord injury, stroke, or simply being too weak from a long hospital stay, you are at risk of getting a pressure sore.

Location, Location, Location

Pressure sores are most common in areas on your body where an object (such as a mattress) compresses skin and the underlying tissues over a bone (such as a hip) in the body. Other factors that contribute to the problem include shearing forces, friction, and moisture. A little pressure and a little of one or more of these other factors will greatly increase your risk of developing a pressure sore. Each of these factors adds to the pressure's already destructive effects. Figure 5 shows common locations where pressure sores may develop.

Pressure

Small blood vessels are called capillaries. In frail or ill people, blood pressures in these capillaries may be much lower than those in young, healthy people. Problems start when the pressure of the force between the surface you are lying on and the bones underneath is greater than the pressure of the blood in the capillaries.

Think of water moving through a garden hose, then imagine what happens when you put your foot on the hose. If the pressure you are applying on the hose is more than the pressure of the water moving through the hose, the water stops moving through the hose. The same concept can be applied for blood moving through capillaries.

If the pressure continues long enough, capillaries collapse and toxins accumulate. Cells in nearby muscle and tissues begin to die. Muscle and fat are more vulnerable to interruptions in blood flow than skin. Consequently, by the time warning signs appear on the skin (such

---

Myth: Pressure sores can be caused by falls.
Truth: Injuries and breaks in the skin caused by falls should heal quickly. A pressure sore starts because of immobility or other causes.

Regularly check your skin in these
places for redness or skin breakdown.

(if you have a wound that is not in
one of these spots, the cause of the
wound is not likely a pressure sore)

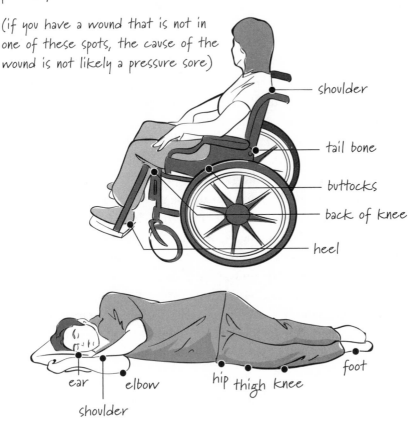

shoulder

tail bone

buttocks

back of knee

heel

ear | elbow | hip thigh knee | foot

shoulder

Figure 5: Pressure points.

as redness and skin breakdown), the underlying muscle and fat have
probably suffered significant damage. So once you see the problem,
some damage has already been done. If you've noticed something that
sounds like this kind of damage, contact your physician immediately.

The pressure involved in creating a pressure sore comes from not
one but two sources. When blood vessels, muscle, and skin are compressed between a bone and an external surface—a bed or chair, for

instance—pressure is exerted on the tissues from both the external surface and the bone. In effect, the external surface produces pressure and the bone produces counterpressure. Although the pressure affects all tissues between these two points, tissues closest to the bone suffer the greatest damage.

When the body's weight is resting on a small area, the pressure is very high. If you make the resting area bigger, there is less pressure over that area. Think of a group of gymnasts who want to reach the top of the gymnasium by climbing on each others' shoulders. If a single person supported the group, that would be a lot of pressure for the bottom person because the weight would be distributed over a small area. However, if the gymnasts were to stack themselves in the shape of a pyramid, the weight would be more evenly distributed, and consequently less pressure would be exerted on the person at the base. Therefore, bony prominences such as your hip bones, because they have a small surface area, are particularly susceptible to pressure sores. However, they aren't the only areas at risk. Sores can develop on any soft tissue when it is put under pressure for a long time.

In people who have normal sensation and mobility, pressure that occurs over time causes a growing discomfort that prompts them to

 Pressure and Hard Surfaces

Many people ask: "How hard does a surface have to be for a pressure sore to occur?" More important than the surface, however, is the length of time the pressure is applied. Low pressure for long periods is far more damaging than high pressure for short periods. Sitting for several hours a day in a chair that does not have a proper pressure-relieving cushion actually causes more problems than sitting for a very short time on a surface that is rock hard.

change position before tissue damage and ulceration occurs. In fact, most people shift position every fifteen minutes, without even being aware of it! This is why you do not get pressure sores from sleeping— you shift your weight continuously through the night. If you do not have normal sensation (e.g., paraplegia) and have decreased mobility, you may not feel the discomfort from any pressure, and as a result don't naturally shift position often enough.

Although pressure sores can result from one period of sustained pressure, they are more likely to result from repeated high pressure episodes without enough time to recover in between. This was the case with Mr. H, the patient in our clinic who was using a new lift repeatedly through the day. The lift exerted high pressure around his hip bones, and there was not enough time for that tissue to recover.

Shear

Shearing force is the mechanical force that occurs when two side by side surfaces move in opposite directions (such as skin and the underlying soft tissue and muscles). It runs parallel to an area of skin, rather than perpendicular (like pressure does).

Shear is most likely to develop during repositioning or when a person slides down the bed after being placed with their back perpendicular to their legs. Elevating the head of the bed increases shear and pressure in the tailbone area because gravity pulls the body down, but the skin on the back resists the motion due to friction between the skin and the sheets. The result is that the skeleton (and attached tissues) actually slides beneath the skin, generating shearing (rubbing) between the tissues under the skin. The force can be strong enough to block or tear blood vessels.

Shearing force reduces the length of time that skin and tissues can survive pressure before a lack of oxygen develops (that is, your skin and tissues won't be able to withstand immobility and pressure if there is also a rubbing, shearing force during transfers). If there is a high level of shearing force, the blood flow to an area of skin can be blocked by half the amount of pressure normally required, creating sores much sooner.

Sores on the tailbone shaped like triangles or sores with deep tunneling are mostly due to shearing forces.

Friction

Friction occurs when one surface moves across another surface—for example, when your skin slides across a bed sheet. A skinned knee is an example of a wound caused by friction.

You are at particularly high risk for tissue damage due to friction if you have uncontrollable movements or spastic conditions, wear braces, prostheses, or appliances that rub against the skin, and are older than

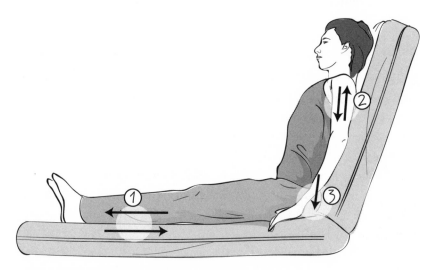

① sheets rubbing against your skin

② skin rubbing against your muscles and bones as you slide down in bed (this is especially bad if the head of the bed is nearly upright)

③ pressure of your tailbone against the bed

Figure 6: Forces in a bed that can cause a pressure sore.

age sixty. Friction is also a problem if you have trouble lifting yourself during repositioning. As shown in Figure 6, rubbing against the sheets (during transfers or spasms, for example) can result in a wound due to friction. Elevating the head of your bed too far upright generates friction between your skin and the bed sheets as gravity pulls your body down. As your skeleton moves inside your skin, friction and shear combine to increase the risk of tissue damage in the tailbone area.

There are ways to minimize friction, however. Dry lubricants such as cornstarch and adherent dressings with slippery backings can help reduce problems associated with friction.

Moisture

Too much moisture (for example, from sweat, wound drainage, urine, or stool) can saturate your skin. Another word for the condition of waterlogged skin is maceration*. Maceration contributes to pressure sore formation by softening the tissues. Macerated skin erodes more easily, degenerates, and eventually rubs off. Damp skin also sticks to bed linens more easily, so the effects of any shear or friction are made much worse. In fact, moist skin is five times more likely to develop sores than dry skin.

Pressure Sore Stages

Not all pressure sores are alike. The National Pressure Ulcer Advisory Panel (NPUAP) categorizes (or assigns stages to) pressure sores. Your wound specialist will determine the stage of your wound and treat it accordingly.

> *Deep tissue injury*: A purple area of skin or a blood-filled blister can mean deep damage underneath the skin. Deep tissue injury may be difficult to detect in individuals with dark skin, as the skin's color can mask the signs of tissue damage. Deep tissue injury is much like an iceberg—what you can see at the surface is a small part, but the area that you cannot see is much bigger. As there is a larger portion of damage that

cannot be seen, a pressure sore may rapidly develop in that area.

Stage I: This is tricky: a stage I pressure sore isn't actually an open sore. There is no break in the skin. It is an area of persistent redness in people with light skin or persistent red, blue, or purple in people with darker skin. It is an area that is at high risk of breaking down further, so take action now to prevent further problems.

Stage II: A stage II pressure ulcer is a superficial wound that looks like a scrape or a blister.

Stage III: A stage III pressure ulcer is a full-thickness wound with tissue damage that can extend deeply. The ulcer presents as a deep crater.

Stage IV: A stage IV ulcer involves full-thickness skin loss with extensive damage to muscle, bone, and supporting structures (such as tendons and joint).

Am I at Risk for Developing a Pressure Sore?

Immobility is the most important risk factor for developing a pressure sore. Other important risk factors include: poor nutrition, obesity, advanced age, incontinence, infection, low blood pressure, and altered consciousness. All these risk factors are discussed further below. If you

Table 1. Pressure Ulcer Risk Factors

- Is your mobility impaired?
- Do you have a spinal cord injury?
- Do you have advanced multiple sclerosis?
- Do you have advanced Parkinson's disease?
- Do you have advanced Alzheimer's dementia?
- Do you live in a nursing home?
- Are you an inpatient in a hospital or will you be admitted at some point soon?

have one or more of these risk factors, you need to be checked regularly for early signs of pressure sores.

Generally, the longer you're in the hospital or nursing home, the greater your chances for developing a pressure sore. However, you also have a high likelihood of developing a pressure sore within the first two weeks of admission to a long-term care facility. Your medical team and loved ones should check your skin regularly during all high-risk times.

Immobility

Immobility is the greatest risk factor for pressure sore development. Being able to move in response to being uncomfortable from too much pressure is very important for preventing pressure sores; therefore, if you are not able to move, you are much more likely to develop sores.

Nutrition

Proper nutrition is essential to keep your skin healthy (see Chapter 32).

Obesity

If you are very overweight, you may be at risk for pressure sore development for several reasons:

- Your nutritional status may not be good.
- You may be prone to developing protein malnutrition even though you may have excess body fat storage.
- You have more fat tissue, which has decreased blood flow compared to other tissues in the body.
- It may be challenging to change position or move.
- Your skin folds may be moist, which can lead to pressure ulcers. These areas can be a breeding ground for bacteria, which then can lead to fungal infections.

We discuss obesity and skin in greater detail in Chapter 26.

Advancing Age

The risk of developing pressure sores increases with age because aging affects all aspects of healing. As skin gets older, it becomes more fragile as blood flow decreases and skin layers adhere less securely to one another. Older adults have less lean body mass and less tissue under the skin cushioning bony areas. Therefore, they are more likely to suffer skin and tissue damage due to friction, shear, and pressure. Many older adults may also have other risk factors for pressure ulcer development, including poor nutrition (see Chapters 22 and 23).

Incontinence

Incontinence increases a person's exposure to moisture and, over time, increases risk of skin breakdown. Both urine and stool which stay on the skin for a long period of time irritate the skin and make it more susceptible to bacterial infection. Stool probably causes more skin damage than urine does.

Infection

Pressure on the skin and tissues may increase bacterial growth in that area of your body. In areas where there is a loss of sensation (as in people with a spinal cord injury or diabetic neuropathy), your body may not be able to fight infection. This may explain why people with loss of sensation are more at risk of developing infection in pressure sores.

Blood Pressure

Low blood pressure usually means that less oxygen is being delivered to the skin and tissues. When blood pressure is low, the body conserves oxygen by moving blood away from the vascular system that serves the skin and toward vital organs such as the heart and lungs. High blood pressure has dangerous effects on your health too, so it is important to talk with your health-care team about the range of blood pressure that is safest for you.

We talked with Mrs. E and her family and helped them develop strategies to take off some of the pressure while she was sleeping. This included changing her mattress and using pillows. She agreed to take antibiotics to fight her infection. We also suggested she use a different dressing that was more absorbent. After about two weeks, her pain had decreased. It took several months, but Mrs. E's wound healed, and she now enjoys playing with her grandchildren again and takes extra care when there is ice on the ground.

6
Prevention Is Always Best

Once you suspect that you may be at risk for developing pressure sores, you are already one step ahead of the game. Now you can take action to prevent them from occurring.

Support aids, cushions, and beds play an important role in pressure ulcer prevention (for more information on beds and cushions, see Chapter 7). Proper nutrition, including a balanced diet and maintaining a healthy body weight, is also important for preventing and healing pressure ulcers (see Chapter 32). Common problems with skin that can make wounds more likely to occur, or keep wounds from healing properly, are discussed in Chapter 35.

Managing Pressure

It can be challenging to control the amount of pressure your skin is exposed to, especially if you have limited mobility. Managing the amount and duration of pressure is the most important part of preventing pressure sores from developing.

Frequent and careful repositioning of your immobile loved one helps him or her avoid the damaging pressure that leads to skin damage that can eventually cause a sore to form.

Encouraging Mobility

Physical activity decreases your risk of pressure sore development. Encourage activity as much as you can. Start with a small goal—help your loved one out of bed and into a chair. Make sure to speak to your health-care team so you know how to lift and transfer him or her properly, without injuring either one of you. Once he or she can tolerate more activity, move on to bigger goals—help him or her walk around the room and then down the hall. *Always have this approved by a physical therapist and/or occupational therapist to ensure your loved one's safety.*

The Right Way to Reposition

Any time you reposition your loved one, look for telltale areas of reddened skin, and make sure the new position does not place weight on these areas.

If the affected area is on an arm or leg, use pillows to support the limb to reduce the pressure. Avoid raising the head of the bed more than thirty degrees to prevent tissue damage due to friction and shearing force.

POSITIONING A PERSON IN BED

A person who is vulnerable for pressure sores should lie in bed in such a way as to minimize the chance of developing pressure ulcers

How often should I check my skin (or that of a loved one) who is at high risk for pressure sores?

If at home or in a nursing home: every three days
If in a hospital: every twenty-four hours

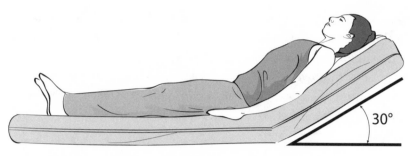

Keep the head of the bed at 30 degrees or
lower (except while eating, when the head of
the bed should be raised higher)

When you are on your side, use a
pillow or other bolster to tilt you
over at about 30 degrees.
Lying too far on your side means
you will be directly over your
hip bone, where pressure ulcers
can occur more easily.

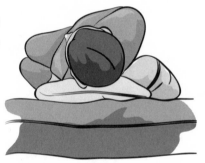

Figure 7: How to lie in bed to help prevent pressure sores.

(Figure 7). When the person is on his or her side, never allow weight
to rest directly on the bony area of the hip. Instead, rest weight on the
buttocks and use a pillow or foam wedge to help the person stay in that
position. This position ensures that no pressure is placed on the bony
area of hip or the tailbone. Also, placing a pillow between the knees
or ankles minimizes the pressure exerted when one limb lies on top of
the other.

It is important to *protect the heels* from pressure, although this
can be difficult. Even when heels are being supported by specially designed cushions, reducing the pressure on heels to allow for perfect
blood flow is almost impossible. Instead, lift the person's leg off of
the bed and put a pillow under their calves. This allows for the heels

to be suspended in a comfortable position. Keeping the heels off of the hard surface maintains the blood flow to the heel. Remember to take care to avoid permanent knee contraction. This can be done by frequent repositioning—including doing passive range of motion exercises of your loved one's legs. A physical therapist or occupational therapist can be your best friend when it comes to teaching you these techniques.

POSITIONING A PERSON WHO IS SEATED

The right posture and alignment helps to ensure that the weight of the person's body is distributed as evenly as possible (Figure 8). For some people, sitting straight up tends to focus all of their weight on the relatively small surface area over the ischial tuberosities (also called "sit" bones), and may increase the risk of pressure ulcers in these areas. For other people, reclining may be more likely to cause pressure ulcers than sitting straight up. Whatever position is better for you, it is still important to reposition frequently. Staying in one position too long, no matter how ideal the positioning, can lead to pressure sores.

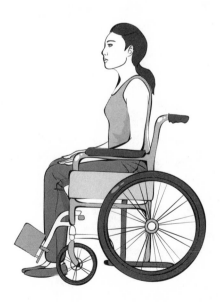

Figure 8: The right posture to help prevent pressure sores.

Maintain good posture. Proper posture alone can significantly reduce your risk of pressure ulcers.

- Sit with your back straight and against the back of the chair
  and arms supported by the arms of the chair. This position
  distributes weight evenly over the available body surface area.
- Keep your feet flat on the floor to protect your heels from pressure. This position distributes the weight of your legs over the
  largest available surface area—the soles.
- Don't slouch. Slouching causes shearing and friction, and
  places pressure on the tailbone.
- Keep your knees slightly apart to prevent knees and ankles
  from rubbing together and causing sores.

Put your feet up. If your loved one likes to use an ottoman or footstool, check to see if his or her knees are positioned above hip level.
If so, it means that his or her weight has shifted from the back of the
thighs to the bony hips. The same problem—knees above hips—can
occur if the chair itself is too short for the patient. In this case, recommend that he or she use a different footstool or chair.

If you use a wheelchair and are able to shift your weight somewhat, it can be enormously helpful to shift your weight from
one side of the buttocks to the other every fifteen minutes or so.
Leaning forward slightly and leaning backward slightly can also
help rearrange weight distribution. These are all frequent adjust-
ments that most people with normal mobility do naturally on a
regular basis.

Reposition. If you are at high risk for developing a pressure sore, you should reposition yourself every fifteen minutes while sitting, if you can. People with spinal cord injuries can perform wheelchair pushups to intermittently relieve pressure on the buttocks and sacrum; however, this requires a fair amount of upper body strength. Some people are not able to use their arms in this way. In this case your wound team, physical therapist, or occupational therapist should be able to recommend exercises and movements that are within the range of your ability.

Managing Incontinence

If you have problems controlling your bowels and/or bladder, you need to carefully monitor your skin to make sure no problems are developing. There are specific steps you can take to prevent skin damage caused by too much moisture, skin irritation, or infection. Three types of aids can help you manage incontinence: incontinence collectors, incontinence undergarments, and mattress/cushion pads and topical barriers.

Incontinence Collectors

- Condom catheters can help manage urinary incontinence in men (similar but less effective devices exist for women).
- Fecal incontinence collectors come with an attached, drainable pouch.
- Collectors need to be changed on a regular schedule and whenever a leak is detected.

The Pros and Cons of Catheters for Incontinence

Pro: Very effective in keeping you clean and dry.
Cons: They increase your risk of a bladder infection; they can restrict your movement; and they are often uncomfortable.

Incontinence Undergarments and Mattress/Cushion Pads

- Pads (including disposable absorbent gel pads and reusable, washable cloth pads) wick moisture away from your skin. Disposable gel pads are much more absorbent and effective than other options, while the cloth pads are the least expensive.
- Change undergarments and mattress/cushion pads promptly when they get wet, so check them frequently. Keep as clean and dry as possible.

Topical Skin Barriers

Barriers are items than you can apply directly on the skin that protect the skin from urine or stool. One type of barrier is similar to a liquid plastic, which comes in a spray-on form or as a disposable wipe. As they dry, these products form a strong barrier on the skin's surface that isn't easily washed off during normal cleaning. Other barriers include pastes, such as zinc oxide (which is often used on a baby's bottom) or petroleum jelly, both of which can protect your skin quite effectively.

What Else Can You Do?

In order to prevent and treat pressure ulcers, you need to understand what your wound team has suggested, and be physically and financially capable of carrying it out at home. Therefore, you need to discuss with your wound team the preferences and lifestyles of you and your family as they may affect your wound care. You and your team should discuss how to prevent pressure ulcers and what to do when they occur. You should discuss repositioning and be shown how to achieve positions that allow for the weight to be redistributed as evenly as possible (see "The Right Way to Reposition" earlier in this chapter). You should be aware of the types of devices available to help maintain these positions and make the person most comfortable. Your wound specialist should also know where you can obtain the devices.

You or your family member should be shown how to examine your back, and any other areas you can't easily see, using a mirror. It

Pressure Ulcer Dos and Don'ts

With proper skin care and frequent position changes, you and your caregivers can keep the skin healthy—a crucial element in pressure ulcer prevention. Here are some important dos and don'ts:

DO . . .

- Change position at least once every two hours while reclining. Follow a schedule. Lie on your right side, then your left side, then your back, then your stomach (if possible). Use pillows and pads for support. Make small turns between the two-hour changes.
- Regularly check your skin for signs of pressure ulcers. Use a mirror to check areas you can't inspect directly, such as the shoulders, tailbone, hips, elbows, heels, and back of the head. Report any breaks in the skin or changes in skin temperature to your wound specialist.
- Follow the prescribed exercise program, including range-of-motion exercise every eight hours or as recommended.
- Eat a well-balanced diet, drink lots of fluids, and strive to maintain your recommended weight.
- Use oil-free lotions.

DON'T . . .

- Use commercial soaps or skin products that dry or irritate your skin.
- Sleep on wrinkled bed sheets or tuck your covers tightly into the foot of your bed (for more information, see Chapter 7).
- Use doughnut-shaped supports or ring cushions.

is important to inspect your skin over bony prominences for pressure-related damage every day. This way you can address problems with pressure as soon as they develop and before significant damage occurs.

If you need to apply dressings at home, it is important to find out exactly where you can purchase supplies. Most medical supply stores or home health agencies stock several wound care products, but check with your wound team to ensure that what they are ordering is readily available. It is also just as important to make sure you understand the proper ways to apply and remove your dressings. For example, some adhesive bandages can damage tissues if removed improperly. Also, dressings sometimes come off due to excessive moisture or wear, and it is essential that you or your family member knows how to dress the wound on your own.

Pressure ulcers should be reassessed weekly by your wound team or other health-care provider. Evidence of healing, if enough blood flow is present, should be apparent in about two to four weeks. If there's no evidence of this, and you have been following your wound team's recommendations regarding nutrition, repositioning, use of support surfaces, and wound dressings, it is time to reevaluate the plan. Discuss this with your wound specialist on your next clinic visit.

7
Beds and Cushions
Expensive Is Not Always Best

The variety of products geared to effective prevention and treatment of your pressure ulcer can be overwhelming. Options to choose from include special beds, mattresses, and seating options that now use foams, gels, water, and air as cushions. The more you and your loved ones learn about your options, the better prepared you all are to give the best care possible.

Beds and Mattresses

Horizontal support surfaces include beds, mattresses, and mattress overlays. These products use foams, gels, water, or air to reduce pressure while you lie in bed.

Specialty beds, such as rotating beds, relieve pressure by rotating your body or helping to lift your body to reduce the risk of friction and shear. However, these mattresses are expensive and not often readily available for home use.

Low-air-loss and *high-air-loss* mattresses are specialized support devices that pass air over the skin. These mattresses promote evaporation and are especially useful when skin is too wet. However, there is risk of dehydration with the use of high-air-loss mattresses, because the body may lose more water than it should due to this evaporation. *Water* mattresses and some *air* mattresses attempt to evenly distribute pressure under your body. Water mattresses use a gentle wave

Selecting a Bed or Chair

Before selecting a bed or chair, answer the following questions:

- Where are the areas that need pressure relief? How much pressure needs to be relieved?
- Are you and your loved one likely to actually use it? Is it comfortable?
- Is the product suitable for your living arrangement? Does it fit into your home/living environment?
- Consider a product's noise factor—for example, will the pump of the mattress disrupt your sleep?
- Does the product require maintenance, and how much?
- How much does the mattress cost, and how much are the extra costs (e.g., power, linen)?
- Would costs be better spent on another part of the treatment plan (e.g., a lift rather than a bed, if transfers are the major problem)?

motion to maintain even distribution of pressure. Several types of air mattresses alternately inflate and deflate tubes within the mattress to distribute pressure.

Mattress overlays are surfaces that are placed on top of a mattress in order to reduce pressure. The most common mattress overlays used in pressure ulcer prevention are foam, air, and gel overlays. Foam overlays should be at least 3 inches (7.6 cm) thick for the average person; thicker is even better. Although 2-inch (5.1 cm) foam overlays may add comfort, they are not enough to prevent pressure ulcers if you are at risk. Solid foam is preferable to the convoluted ("egg-crate") version. Higher-quality foam and high-density foam will last longer and be more effective.

You want to avoid "bottoming out" to the mattress below. If your weight completely compresses a mattress overlay, the overlay is not helping. To make sure that you or your loved one isn't "bottoming out" on the overlay, hand check whenever a new overlay is put into service or if you suspect an overlay is breaking down. To hand check an overlay, slide one hand—palm up and fingers outstretched—between the mattress overlay and the mattress. If you can feel the person's body

Taking a Load Off: Terms for Pressure-Reducing Devices

These special pads, mattresses, and beds help relieve pressure when you or your loved one is confined to one position for long periods.

Air-fluidized bed: Airflow in the mattress helps to support the individual, and this reduces shearing and friction.

Alternating-pressure air mattress: Alternating deflation and inflation of mattress tubes change areas of pressure.

Foam mattress or pads: Must be at least 3 to 4 inches (8–10 cm) thick to adequately cushion skin and minimize pressure.

Foot cradle: A foot cradle lifts the bed linens to relieve pressure over the feet.

Gel pads: Gel pads spread pressure over a wide surface area.

Low-air-loss beds: Inflated air cushions adjust for optimal pressure relief, automatically adjusting for body size.

Mechanical lifting devices: Lift sheets and other mechanical lifting devices prevent shearing by lifting you rather than dragging you across the bed.

Padding: Pillows, towels, and soft blankets, when positioned properly, can reduce pressure in body hollows.

Water mattress or pads: A wave effect provides even distribution of the patient's body weight.

through the overlay, replace the overlay with a thicker one or add more air to the mattress.

Bottom line: For people at home who are at high risk for developing a pressure sore (for example, who have limited mobility), or who have a minor, superficial pressure sore, a proper mattress overlay is usually enough. For people with deep pressure ulcer, a more specialized bed may be necessary.

Speak to your wound team. Whichever support surface you choose, however, it cannot replace the need to change position frequently and properly.

 How to Sit Safely

Everyone who spends time in a wheelchair should be evaluated by an occupational therapist or physical therapist who is experienced in seating assessments.

- Make sure the cushion is positioned correctly (contours facing up, pummel at the front)
- Make sure the cushion is properly maintained (Figure 9)
- Shift your weight (from side to side or lean forward)

Seating should be reevaluated by an occupational therapist or a physical therapist every two to three years or with any one of the following:

- Development of redness
- Development of a new pressure sore
- Increased use of the wheelchair
- Change in your physical status
- Inability to maintain upright posture
- Cushion appears worn or develops leaks

Seating

If you use a wheelchair or spend a lot of time in a regular chair, you need a specialized seat cushion. Often, a foam cushion that is 3–4 inches (7.5–10 cm) thick is enough. If you use a wheelchair, you should have your chair checked at least every two years in a wheelchair clinic. Many wheelchair-seating clinics now use computers to create custom seating systems tailored to fit the needs of each person. For those with spinal cord injuries, the selection of wheelchair seating is based on pressure evaluation, lifestyle, postural stability, continence, and cost. Custom seats and cushions are more expensive; however, in this case, the added expense is justifiable. People who use wheelchairs for most

Make sure you inflate your seating cushion properly

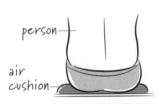

person—

air
cushion—

wrong: the cushion is underinflated, so there is not enough air between your backside and the chair. The cushion has "bottomed out."

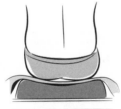

wrong: anything (even a bedsheet) placed between you and the cushion makes the cushion less effective. You cannot sink down properly into the cushion.

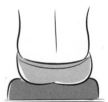

correct! The cushion forms around the shape of your back-side, so you are "floating" in the cushion. You can check to make sure the cushion is properly inflated by having a friend slide their hand under the cushion while you are sitting on it–their hand should easily slide under.

Figure 9: Make sure your seat cushion is properly maintained.

or all the time should replace seat cushions as soon as their current one begins to deteriorate.

Be informed, but also be careful. Using special cushions and mattresses can give you a false sense of security. It is important to remember that as helpful as these devices may be, *they are not substitutes for shifting positions regularly*, regardless of the equipment used. The person should change positions more often if she or he is more vulnerable to developing pressure sores. A cushion or mattress can never replace good care.

Repositioning

Repositioning is just as important when you are sitting as when you are lying down. If you require assistance with repositioning, various devices are available, including lifts, overhead frames, trapezes, walkers, and canes. These devices can help you reposition yourself as necessary.

Hoyer lifts and trapeze bars, for people who are strong enough to lift themselves, can help reduce shear and friction when you transfer between bed to chair and vice versa. These devices allow you to be lifted straight up and away from surfaces, instead of pulled along surfaces and potentially damaging your skin.

Initial use of these devices should always be under the supervision of a physical or occupational therapist. If you start to see a sore developing that you think might be related to how you transfer from the chair or bed, have the therapist reevaluate the device and your technique. As mentioned in Chapter 5, our patient's lift was not properly fitted, and consequently caused continued pressure to his hip bones, resulting in a pressure sore.

Is Bed Rest Effective Treatment for Pressure Ulcers?

Health-care practitioners have slowly moved away from recommending bed rest (defined as twelve hours a day in bed) for many medical conditions. For example, bed rest for two months was once prescribed routinely for patients after a heart attack.

Some health-care practitioners feel that if a person has a bedsore caused by sitting, then he or she should spend most of their time lying down (that is, not sitting) in order to reduce the pressure on the area, and therefore heal the ulcer faster. However, even if bed rest did speed the healing of pressure sores, bed rest does not result in the best quality of life.

In one study, young healthy persons placed in a simulated hospital room developed confusion after 2.75 hours, and the confusion persisted even after the bed rest was stopped and normal activity resumed. If this can happen to a young healthy person, what must happen to the

Table 2: Managing Pressure Throughout the Day

Surface	Your Best Strategy
General (all surfaces) — bed, wheelchair, commode, toilet seat, kitchen chair, couch, etc.	— Use special support surfaces/cushions (talk to your wound team) — Check skin for areas of breakdown or persistent redness — Try to maximize mobility — Determine other factors contributing to skin breakdown: deal with bowel and urinary incontinence, nutrition
Bed	— Change position (talk to your wound team about how to do this) every two hours if possible
Wheelchair	— Shift weight from one side of the buttocks to the other every fifteen minutes if possible
Transfers	— Talk to a physiotherapist or occupational therapist about the best type of lifting device to use. Everyone is different! Lifts that are safe for some people may cause pressure and shear for you.
Commode	— Add a pressure-reducing material to commodes — If the pressure on a bath seat cannot be reduced to a safe level, sponge bathing may be the best option

frail older adult who lies in bed day after day? In additional to confusion, depression is another problem that can occur with prolonged
bed rest.

Alternatives to bed rest include improving nutrition, repositioning, and reducing friction and shear during transfers. Table 2 lists various strategies to manage pressure throughout the day so you can sit
up rather than spend all day in bed. These steps allow you to maintain quality of life while preventing or promoting healing of pressure
sores.

PART THREE

Foot Wounds

Diabetes and Beyond

If you have diabetes, you may be prone to developing foot ulcers due to nerve damage (neuropathy*) and poor blood circulation. You are at even higher risk if your blood sugar is often too high or too low. In addition to foot ulcers, people with diabetes can also develop wounds in other parts of their body (we discuss these nonfoot wounds in Chapter 16).

Good diabetes control may help prevent all of these potentially serious problems or at least make them less severe. It is never too early or too late to optimize your blood sugar control. Better control of blood sugar results in a lower risk of foot ulcers, and in faster healing if they do occur.

The two types of diabetes mellitus that occur in people who are not pregnant are known as type 1 and type 2.

Type 1 diabetes (formerly called juvenile diabetes or insulin-dependent diabetes) is often, but not always, first diagnosed in children or young adults. In this type of diabetes, the pancreas no longer makes insulin.

Type 2 diabetes (formerly called adult-onset or noninsulin-dependent diabetes) can occur at any age, and is the most common form of diabetes. In this type of diabetes, the body is resistant to insulin; that is, the fat, muscle, and liver cells do not use insulin properly. Eventually, the pancreas stops producing enough insulin.

One of the functions of insulin is to transport glucose (sugar) from the bloodstream into cells, where it is used as fuel or stored. If there isn't enough working insulin (because of either type 1 or type 2 diabetes), glucose doesn't get transported into cells and instead stays in the bloodstream. When the blood glucose level starts to get very high, symptoms such as sweatiness and dizziness appear. If your blood glucose stays high for months or years, damage to the blood vessels and nerves can occur. Figure 10 shows the physiological consequences of this damage.

In addition to nerve damage from abnormal blood sugars, another common problem in people with diabetes is poor blood flow to the feet. This poor blood flow can result because of damage to the blood vessels from long-term high blood sugars. Poor blood flow can increase

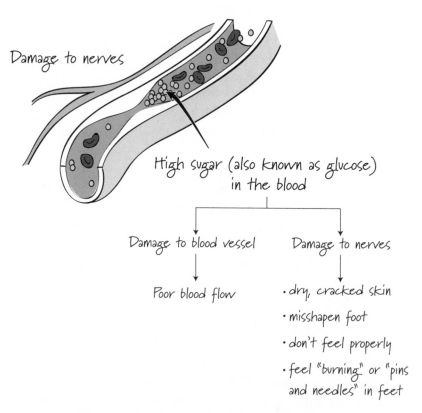

Figure 10: What happens to the blood vessels in diabetes.

your risk of developing ulcers and can also slow the healing process for existing ulcers. Additionally, poor blood flow can slow the distribution of any antibiotics you may take to treat an infected foot ulcer.

Diabetes Facts

- Diabetes is the seventh-leading cause of death in the United States.
- Approximately 20.8 million people (7 percent of the population) have diabetes.
- Each year, more than 1.5 million new cases of diabetes are diagnosed.
- Diabetes occurs most frequently in African Americans, Latinos, Asian Americans, and Native Americans, with middle-age and older adults at highest risk (see Chapter 25).
- About 15 percent of all people with diabetes will develop foot ulcers.
- Men with diabetes are 1.4 to 2.7 times more likely to need an amputation than women with diabetes.

8
The Foot Wound That
Doesn't Hurt

Mr. A is a thirty-two-year-old man. In his early twenties, when he learned that he had diabetes, he became very angry. He then became depressed and did not take his insulin as it was prescribed. Two months ago he developed a foot ulcer. Because his blood sugars had not been steady, he had developed neuropathy and could not feel the ulcer, and only discovered it when he found blood on his sock and took a close look at his foot. After a month, the wound was not healing. He went to see his family doctor, who referred Mr. A to our clinic.

When you have diabetes, wounds can happen for many reasons. Nerve damage, high pressure and friction (for example, shoes that rub because they do not fit properly), and poor circulation can cause foot ulcers.

Diabetic Neuropathy (Nerve Damage)

Neuropathy is the main reason that ulcers develop in people with diabetes. Neuropathy is a nerve disorder that results in impaired function in the skin or muscle served by the affected nerves. In diabetes, neuropathy may be caused by direct nerve damage or poor blood circulation leading to nerve damage.

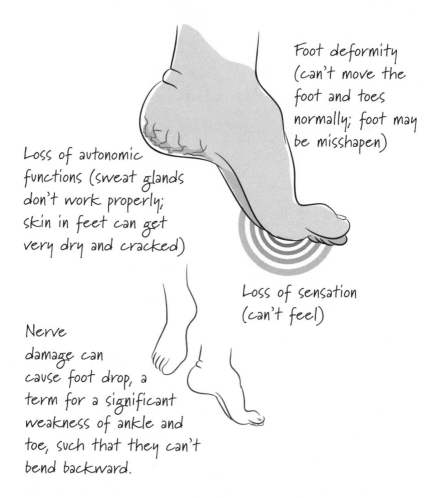

Foot deformity (can't move the foot and toes normally; foot may be misshapen)

Loss of autonomic functions (sweat glands don't work properly; skin in feet can get very dry and cracked)

Loss of sensation (can't feel)

Nerve damage can cause foot drop, a term for a significant weakness of ankle and toe, such that they can't bend backward.

Figure 11: The consequences of neuropathy (nerve damage) can be severe.

People with diabetes tend to have poor blood circulation due to thickening in the tiny blood vessels. The thicker the wall of the blood vessels, the less blood can pass through the vessel, which means that the area, and the nerve, where the vessel leads also gets less blood.

When damage to multiple types of nerves occurs, your risk of developing foot ulcers goes up dramatically. Figure 11 shows the consequences of neuropathy.

Figure 12 shows the areas of the foot where ulcers are most prone to developing. For example, many people with diabetes have damage to three types of nerves in the foot that can result in:

- Loss of sensation (can't feel)
- Foot deformity (can't move the foot and toes normally; foot may be misshapen)
- Loss of autonomic functions (sweat glands don't work properly; skin in feet can get very dry and cracked)

Usually, the longest nerves in the body are affected first. Therefore, neuropathy usually starts in the feet, but if damage continues it can spread toward the knees and even include the hands.

Diabetes is not the only cause of neuropathy. Some other common causes are chemotherapy, vitamin B12 deficiency, and alcohol abuse. In

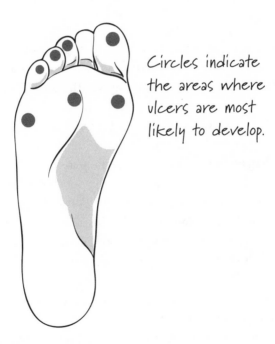

Circles indicate the areas where ulcers are most likely to develop.

Figure 12: Foot ulcers.

many people, the cause of neuropathy is unknown (idiopathic). People who have neuropathy *from any cause* may have feet like those of someone with diabetes. They are at high risk of developing ulcers and need to take very good care of their feet.

Loss of Sensation

Loss of feeling can paradoxically create a burning or "pins and needles" sensation that may worsen at night. As the ability to feel decreases, risk of foot injury increases because you may not sense things (such as pain and pressure) that normally would warn you of impending danger. For example, some people with severe nerve damage can step on a needle and, if barefoot, not even know it. Anything from stepping on something sharp to wearing shoes that are too tight can result in foot injury because you may not feel the damage happening.

Foot Deformity

Nerve damage can cause muscles in the feet to weaken, which causes a condition called foot drop* (significant weakness of ankle and toe, such that it is difficult to flex the foot upward). This nerve damage can also lead to structural deformities resulting in increased arch height and clawed toes. The risk of ulcer development is high for the top (upper surfaces) of clawed toes, especially if you have poorly fitted shoes. Structural changes in the foot cause the fat pad that normally protects the ball of your foot to move, so the ball of your foot experiences more pressure and therefore can develop ulcers. These changes can increase your risk of stumbling or falling and further damaging the foot.

If you have loss of sensation plus weakened, thin bones, the bones can have tiny breaks that you may not even feel: this condition is called a Charcot foot*. Proper footwear is important to prevent worsening damage. If proper footwear isn't worn, over time, the tiny breaks in the bones continue and result in the collapse of the midfoot into a rocker bottom deformity. This means the shape of your foot changes to look like the bottom of a rocking chair, which is the opposite of the normal shape of the foot. This rocker bottom area is at high risk for developing ulcers. Ulcers that occur in this area heal more slowly than ulcers that occur on the balls of your feet.

Autonomic Neuropathy

Autonomic neuropathy means a disruption in the nerves that control your sweat glands in your feet. When sweat glands malfunction, the skin on your feet dries and cracks. If these cracks are deep, the risk of infection rises. If your blood sugar control is very poor, autonomic neuropathy can be severe. In this case, it can result in uncontrolled blood flow to the feet, which can cause weakness and thinning in your foot and ankle bones.

Causes of Foot Ulcers

Forces that can cause diabetic foot ulcers include pressure, friction, and shear. As with pressure ulcers (see Part II), areas over bony prominences are the most common places for diabetic foot ulcers, including metatarsal heads (the ball of the foot), the big toe, and the heel.

Loss of sensation in the feet places you at increased risk for diabetic foot ulcers caused by pressure—especially if you or a loved one is confined to a bed or wheelchair. Damage can occur in these cases simply by letting your feet rest for too long on a bed or a wheelchair footrest. Loss of sensation prevents a person from feeling the discomfort that results from staying in one position too long.

Although pressure is the major mechanical force at work in the development of diabetic ulcers, it isn't the only one. Friction and shear can cause damage as well. A loose shoe rubbing against the foot or a foot sliding across a bed sheet can cause friction damage. Shearing forces build up when damp skin sticks to a surface while the underlying bone and tissue move. For example, the skin of a sweating foot can cling to a shoe while the underlying tissues slide beneath the skin.

Properly fitting socks and shoes are the key to preventing and treating foot problems caused by pressure, friction, and shear. We discuss these in the next chapter.

Preventing Foot Ulcers

Know the Risk Factors

Identifying your risk factors is an important part of preventing foot ulcers. Loss of sensation is the number one risk factor. Poor blood circulation is another risk factor. Here's a list of some other things that put you at risk if you have diabetes:

- Foot deformity (such as clawed toes or rocker bottom)
- Trauma
- Improperly fitted shoes
- Calluses
- Prolonged, high pressure on your feet
- Limited joint mobility
- Long history of diabetes
- Visual impairment or blindness
- Chronic renal (kidney) disease
- Previous foot ulcer or amputation
- Age (older than sixty-five years)
- High blood pressure
- High blood sugar
- High cholesterol and/or triglycerides
- Obesity

Good Foot Care

If you have diabetes, it is important for you to take excellent care of your feet, including:

- Daily foot examinations
- Skin washing and maintenance techniques
- Keeping toenails trimmed
- Choosing proper shoes and socks (see Chapter 9)

It is important to understand care and prevention of foot ulcers, as well as the importance of controlling diabetes, including the consequences of not controlling it. For example, poorly controlled blood sugar levels can lead to loss of sensation and poor blood flow. In contrast, well managed blood sugar levels reduce severity of loss of sensation. It is never too late to make good choices about your health.

 Proper Foot Care

Here are some tips for proper foot care.

Performing foot hygiene

- Check your feet daily for injury or pressure areas (a long-handled mirror can help to see the bottom and back of your feet)
- Wash your feet with a mild soap and dry thoroughly between your toes
- Check your bath water to make sure it isn't too hot (test the water with your elbow, if able; otherwise, use a thermometer or ask a family member to help)
- Apply a moisturizing cream to prevent dry, cracking skin on your feet and to balance skin pH
- Don't apply moisturizer between the toes
- Cut your toenails off squarely; see a podiatrist if they are deformed and thickened, or if your eyesight is too poor to safely cut your nails
- Never go barefoot; always wear your shoes, even in the house—the risk of injury is too great

(continues)

(continued)

Doing a proper foot exam

No one knows your feet like you do, and you should check your feet daily to make note of any changes. Carefully examine your feet to detect and assess foot ulcers. Check the following high-risk areas of the feet:

- Soles of the toes
- Tips of the toes
- Area between the toes
- Outside area of the bottom of your feet

You are checking for

- Existing ulcers
- Calluses (considered "prewounds")
- Blood blisters (bleeding underneath a callus)
- Redness (a sign of inflammation or infection)
- Skin fissures
- Dry, scaly skin
- Wet, white skin between the toes

The dressings to use on diabetic foot ulcers are discussed further in Chapter 18.

We listened to Mr. A and empathized with his frustrating ordeal. We knew that we would have to build a trusting relationship with Mr. A to help him. We discussed with Mr. A the importance of taking his insulin as prescribed and referred him to a different endocrinologist because he didn't like the one he had. We told him that he had to stay off of his foot and gave him a walking cast. When he came to see us in the clinic he was not wearing his walking cast, and his wound was getting worse because he was still on his feet.

At each appointment we tried to deal with his feelings and help teach him why it was important to follow our suggestions. With time, he got so tired of living with the ulcer that he was ready to do anything. He decided that he would take time off work, take his insulin properly, and wear his walking cast.

Six weeks after he made this decision his wound was healed. He is now very conscientious about caring for his feet.

9
Shoes and Socks
When What You Wear Can Be the Best Medicine

Mrs. Z is a sixty-nine-year-old Italian-born woman. She takes care of everyone in her family, including her husband, kids, grandchildren, and even her older sister. She keeps her house spotless, cooks big family meals each weekend, and is very active in her church. She is a vibrant lady, with a strong Italian accent and a big laugh. She has had diabetes for many years, and developed an ulcer six months ago on the side of her right foot.

When she first came to our clinic, she was very pleasant to talk to and listened to what we had to say—until the topic of shoes came up. Our chiropodist showed her therapeutic footwear that would help with her pressure issues. We told her that she would need to wear her shoes all the time, even in the house, in order to heal her wound and prevent future wounds from occurring. She was visibly upset and said she would never wear those ugly shoes—and never wear dirty shoes on her clean floor.

If you have diabetes (or neuropathy from another cause) and your shoes and socks don't fit properly, serious problems may occur. Wearing appropriate shoes and socks may help avoid potential wounds, and especially if you have had foot wounds in the past, preventing wounds is much easier than treating them. If you already have a wound, the correct socks and shoes are even more important.

Socks

If you have diabetes, your socks should not be too tight, and should not have seams on the inside, where they can rub and put pressure on the skin. If they do have seams, you should turn the socks inside out to wear them. You can also get socks with added padding, which provide some extra cushioning and protection for your feet.

Taking the Pressure Off

The key to foot ulcer prevention if you have neuropathy is relieving the pressure from the soles of the feet. It is the most important thing you can do, not just to prevent ulcers from occurring, but also to help

 Choosing Socks

- Wear white or light-colored socks in order to quickly detect bleeding from trauma
- Wear seamless socks
- Wear socks made out of fiber that can help to wick perspiration away from your feet (such as cotton-blend socks) to prevent moisture buildup
- Use padded socks, specially made for persons with diabetes, for shear and friction control
- Silver ion-lined socks for fungus control are an option if fungal infections are a recurrent problem for you

Get an Expert's Advice

Comfort alone may not be a good guide if you have nerve damage. Just because a shoe feels comfortable doesn't mean it's not squeezing in the wrong places; you just may not know it. Some people with diabetes say they are comfortable in shoes that are too tight; this is because the pressure makes them able to feel their shoes. Have your shoes checked by a podiatrist you trust and make sure that they are comfortable, too.

heal them if they occur. A diabetic foot ulcer will not heal if abnormal pressure on the feet is not reduced or removed. Things that add to abnormally high pressures in certain areas of your foot can include foot deformities, foot injury, or shoes that don't fit well. These all increase your risk of building up damaging pressure and then developing an ulcer in that location.

Because people with diabetic neuropathy can no longer feel the growing discomfort that leads to ulcer formation or that is causing continued pressure on an existing ulcer, relieving foot pressure is very important. There are several ways to relieve this pressure: therapeutic footwear, custom orthotics, walking casts, and sometimes surgery. The first three items mentioned can increase your risk of falling and may not be right for you. Talk to your wound team. If you have had an amputation in the past and wear a prosthesis, it is very important that the prosthesis fits properly, otherwise you may develop a wound or other skin problems at the amputation site (see Chapter 28).

Therapeutic Footwear

If you have recurring ulcers and severe foot deformities, you can greatly benefit from a custom-molded shoe. Figure 13 highlights the special

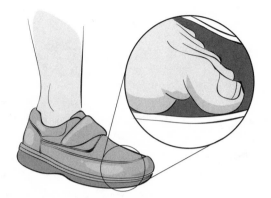

Common design features of therapeutic footwear include a toe box with extra depth and width to accommodate deformities such as clawed toes and bunions.

Figure 13: Therapeutic footwear. Make sure your shoe fits properly!

features of therapeutic footwear. Shoes can vary greatly in price, and expensive is not always better.

Common design features of therapeutic footwear include:

- soft, breathable leather that conforms to foot deformities
- high tops for ankle stability
- rocker soles and bottoms for pressure and pain relief across the plantar metatarsal heads (balls of your feet)
- a toe box with extra depth and width to accommodate deformities such as clawed toes and bunions
- flared lateral soles for stability

Custom Orthotics

Custom orthotics are shoe inserts that serve various functions based on your needs. In general, custom orthotics relieve pressure, reduce shearing force and friction, and cushion the foot against shocks. If necessary, custom orthotics accommodate foot deformities as well.

Choosing Shoes

- Wear well-fitting shoes that are not too tight or loose
- Wear shoes that breathe to reduce moisture buildup and fungal infections
- Wear new shoes for short periods (under one hour) each day initially; gradually increase the time as your feet adjust
- If you have any foot deformities or a history of ulceration, wear professionally fitted shoes
- Wash your shoes, if possible, to destroy microorganisms
- Check your shoes before putting them on to make sure nothing fell in that could cause harm
- Shoes break down quickly; replace your shoes when they are wearing down and not supporting your foot properly

Casts

Casts range from total contact casts to splints and walking casts. A total contact cast is the top of the line in care for uninfected diabetic ulcers on the sole (plantar surface) of the foot. Total contact casts are custom made for you by a health-care professional, typically a physical therapist or orthotist. Inside the cast, padding is fitted over bony areas of the ankle and leg that are at risk for pressure ulcers. A plaster shell reinforced with plaster splints covers the padding. Fiberglass covers the plaster to lend rigidity and additional strength, and the cast includes a sturdy heel for walking. The cast is molded snugly to prevent the foot from sliding inside it. This reduces shearing forces over the plantar surface.

A person with an infected diabetic foot ulcer should not use a total contact cast because a cast makes regular assessment, cleaning, and dressing impossible. In addition, inflammation and swelling can cause a buildup of pressure within the cast and subsequent tissue damage. In the case of infection, a shoe or removable cast that reduces pressure from the ulcer should be used.

Splints and walking casts have cushioned inserts with an outer shell of fiberglass or copolymer. Several splint and walking cast options are available. One advantage of splints and walking casts is that they can be removed easily to allow inspection of the ulcer. In addition, off-loading modifications can be accomplished relatively easily by changing the type of splint or walker in use. However, these devices have disadvantages as well. First and foremost, they do not provide the same degree of pressure and shear relief as a total contact cast. Also, for these therapies to work, you must be committed to using the device—if you choose not to use them regularly, they won't be effective.

Surgery to Reduce Pressure

For some people, surgery can help prevent or treat foot ulcers (see Chapter 21).

Mrs. Z's reaction to having to wear proper footwear is not uncommon. We can understand that wearing therapeutic footwear is not always fashionable or ideal. We also understand that some people never wear shoes at home. We suggested to Mrs. Z that she have a pair of shoes just for her house, which she considered. We also reinforced to her the importance of taking the pressure off of her feet by trying to walk a little less. She reluctantly agreed to our suggestions and wore therapeutic footwear as much as possible.

After three months her wound had healed. We emphasized to her how important it was, now that she had healed, to keep her feet protected by always wearing shoes and looking at her feet every day. Mrs. Z is doing so well that she has never had to come back to our clinic.

PART FOUR

Blood Circulation

Essential for Healing

The word *circulation** refers to the system of blood circulating in your body. The circulatory system (also known as the vascular system) is made up of arteries, veins, capillaries, and lymphatics. Arteries carry blood from the heart to the rest of the body, and veins carry blood from the rest of the body back to the heart (Figure 14). Capillaries connect these two systems. Miles of arteries, capillaries, and veins keep blood circulating from the heart to every part of the body and back again.

Your circulation affects how much blood flow is going to and from the region of your wound. How good your circulation is determines how fast your wound will heal. When you have a lot of swelling (or edema*), this can worsen your circulation. In this section of the book, we discuss how circulation affects your wound and healing, how your health-care team will determine how good your circulation is, and how you can improve your circulation and decrease edema.

Pressure from the beating heart pushes blood away from the heart through the arteries into progressively smaller vessels until they connect with the capillaries, small veins that receive blood and pass it into progressively larger veins on its return trip to the heart. The lymphatic system is a separate system of vessels that collect waste products and deliver them to the venous system.

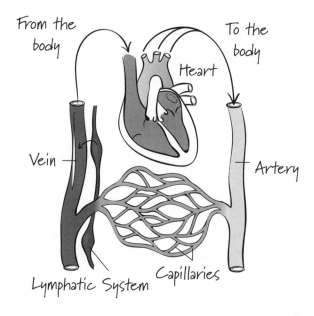

Figure 14: The circulatory system. Good blood flow is essential for healing.

Disorders of the Circulatory System

Diseases that affect the lymphatic vessels, arteries, or veins are known collectively as peripheral vascular disease (PVD). The most common and important type of PVD is peripheral arterial disease, or PAD, which affects about 8 million Americans. It is more common in people who smoke or have diabetes. It also becomes more common as one gets older, and by age sixty-five, about 12 to 20 percent of the population has it. Diagnosis is critical, as people with PAD have four to five times greater risk of heart attack or stroke.

Vascular ulcers are chronic wounds that stem from PVD in the venous, arterial, and lymphatic systems. Venous and arterial ulcers are most common in the distant lower extremities (such as the toes), whereas lymphatic ulcers occur in the arms or the legs. Vascular ulcers differ in appearance and severity, depending on the part of the vascular system that is affected.

The ulcers are only the tip of the iceberg. Your health-care team, and you, must also address the underlying disorder, or the ulcer will not heal. For instance, with venous ulcers, legs must be compressed to encourage fluid back into the veins. With arterial ulcers, arterial blood flow must be restored. Vascular disease can occur all over the body, so your wound team may ask about problems in other areas of the body.

How Good Is Your Circulation?

If you have a wound on your lower leg or foot, your wound team will assess how good your circulation is. They can do this by asking you questions about your medical history, doing a physical exam, performing medical investigations (discussed in Chapter 4), or a combination of these things. Signs of poor circulation are discussed in Chapter 10 ("Venous Wounds") and Chapter 11 ("Arterial Wounds"). The treatment for your leg or foot wound varies depending on whether your circulation is good or poor.

10

Venous Wounds

Dealing with Foot and Leg Wounds if
Your Circulation Is Good

Mr. G is a seventy-seven-year-old retired gentleman with leg ulcers. He had two dogs that he enjoyed walking, but he now finds that his legs swell at the end of the day and cause discomfort. When he was in his thirties he noticed that his legs were developing varicose veins, but until he was in his early seventies, he never developed ulcers. His first ulcer, on the inside of his right ankle, went away by itself after several months. But later he developed another wound in the same place, and this time he was not so lucky: instead of healing, this wound got bigger and bigger. So he started coming to our wound clinic.

When you have good blood flow to the legs and feet, your wounds are most likely due to problems with your veins (for example, varicose veins). Ulcers due to problem veins are called venous ulcers. Venous ulcers cause 70 to 90 percent of all leg ulcers. There are other, unusual causes for leg ulcers, however, so it is important that your wound care team assesses you and diagnoses the exact cause. This chapter explains why venous ulcers develop and discusses how they can be prevented and treated.

Venous Ulcers

Venous ulcers occur on the lower leg and become more common as people get older, especially over the age of sixty. Venous ulcers often occur in people with varicose veins. Varicose veins usually appear as very visible bluish veins that are sometimes winding instead of a straight line. However, you can't always see varicose veins, especially if they are deep. Often you don't even know you have varicose veins until you injure your leg and your wound is very slow to heal. In other words, you might not have known you were at risk for venous ulcers because you weren't able to see the signs of that risk.

Causes of Venous Leg Ulcers

When blood does not come back up through the veins properly, you may develop venous leg ulcers (Figure 15). Veins have a system of cup-shaped valves. The valves function to keep blood flowing in one direction—toward the heart. In most cases, valves that don't work

If you have had any of the following in the past, you may be at risk for having varicose veins and resultant venous leg ulcers:

- Hip or knee surgery
- Blood clots in the leg
- Pregnancies
- Family history of venous insufficiency
- Trauma or damage to the legs (such as broken bones)
- Vein surgery or vein stripping (e.g., vein graft for heart bypass surgery)

Normally, blood in the leg veins flows back from the feet and legs towards the heart. When the valves in these veins are damaged (such as after pregnancy, surgery, blood clots, being overweight or increased age), the blood does not flow back to the heart as quickly. Instead, the blood sits in the lower legs and feet, causing swelling.

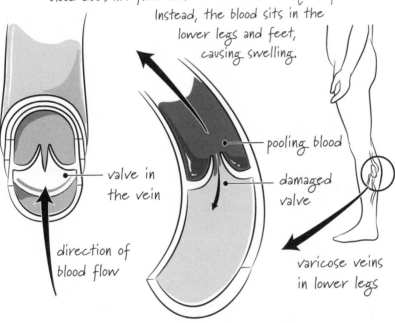

valve in the vein

pooling blood

damaged valve

direction of blood flow

varicose veins in lower legs

Figure 15: Venous leg ulcers. Why varicose veins and venous ulcers occur.

Warning Signs of Possible Venous Leg Ulcers

Initially, problems with your veins don't produce symptoms. You may, however, notice some mild swelling (particularly at the end of the day) and feel a general discomfort or aching in the affected areas.

properly are the cause of venous insufficiency. Valve malfunction may be caused by a blood clot, or stretching of the valves (from any of the risk factors listed in the box).

When the flow of venous blood back up to the heart slows down, blood pools in the veins of the lower legs. Swelling (edema) then develops in the feet, ankles, and (if it is more severe) legs. (For more about swelling see Chapter 12.)

Where Do Venous Ulcers Occur?

Venous ulcers may occur anywhere from the ankle to midcalf; however, they are most common on the inner part of the ankle. The ulcer may extend all the way around the leg and may be red, yellow, black, or a combination of these colors. Most have an irregular shape. The borders may be dry or wet depending on how little or how much drainage there is. You have probably also noticed swelling in the lower leg.

What Do Venous Ulcers Look Like?

When someone has venous insufficiency they usually have changes in the skin color around their ankles. These changes are usually brown in color, surrounding the wound and in the lower leg. This discoloration may have been present even before the ulcer developed. This color change is due to a buildup of deposits under the skin as the red blood cells that have leaked into the skin and tissues break down. Eventually, the skin and tissues underneath can thicken and become fibrotic (scarred). These color changes are permanent, but you can prevent further discoloration by managing the swelling.

Other skin changes that you may see with problems with your veins may include:

- Swelling: This is also called edema and is one of the first signs of venous disease. It may be confined to the foot or the ankle or may involve the entire lower leg. It is usually worse at the end of the day.

- Dry skin and/or itchy skin: This is common. Drainage from the ulcer can irritate the skin and aggravate dryness and itching.

Diagnostic Tests

Often no test is required to diagnose venous disease. However, your doctor may send you for one or more of the following:

> *Venous duplex scanning* is used to assess venous patency (openness, or lack of obstruction) by measuring venous pressures along the leg. This is a noninvasive test.
> *Plethysmography* records changes in the blood volume in the veins. This is a noninvasive test.
> *Venography* involves injecting dye into the vein and taking x-rays. This test is rarely done.

More commonly, your doctor may send you for a test to make sure you have normal arterial blood flow. We describe some of these tests in the section "Diagnostic Tests" in the next chapter. If your arterial blood flow is normal, there is a good chance your ulcers are due to venous disease.

What Can You Do to Improve Your Circulation?

One thing you can do to improve your circulation is to keep moving! Calf muscles have an important role in venous circulation. As calf muscles contract, they squeeze veins in the leg, forcing blood back toward the heart. When they relax, veins in the leg expand and refill with blood. This pumping action is important because about 90 percent of venous blood travels to the heart this way. However, the calf muscles must be active for the calf muscle pump to work. Leg muscle paralysis or prolonged inactivity eliminates the calf muscle pump and inhibits venous blood flow. So sitting for prolonged periods of time can worsen venous insufficiency, whereas walking can improve it.

Is Varicose Vein Surgery a Good Idea?

Veins can be superficial (close to the skin) or deep. Often it is the superficial veins that may not be visually appealing. However, surgery is not always a good idea and can actually increase your risk of developing wounds in the future, particularly if your varicose veins are deep. You may be trading one problem (the cosmetic problem) for one that is worse. Speak to your doctor (or even get a second opinion) before going under the knife.

Controlling edema is the most important goal in managing chronic venous insufficiency (see Chapter 12). Effective treatment of a venous ulcer also involves caring for the wound and managing the underlying venous disease.

You can use the following tips to help promote healing of your venous leg ulcer and reduce your risk of developing new ulcers:

- *Walk* frequently—using your calf muscles aids healing: help your venous ulcers to heal
- *Flex* your feet up and down (as if you were using the gas pedal in a car) frequently when sitting
- *Elevate* your legs as high as is comfortable (above the level of your heart would be best) whenever you sit
- *Compress* your legs with compression stockings as recommended by your wound team
- *Move* your body; don't sit or stand for long periods of time
- *Eat well* and try to achieve your optimal body weight as recommended by your health-care team. Ask for a referral to a nutritionist if you feel you may be overweight. (See Chapter 26 for more information on weight loss.)

After Mr. G's first appointment with us, we sent him for some blood tests, which showed that his blood flow to his legs was adequate. After we explained why compression would be a good treatment, he agreed to give it a try. It was decided that he would receive three layers of compression to the leg that had the wound. On the other leg, he would wear compression stockings to prevent other wounds from forming. Some people are really bothered by the compression the first time they put it on, but Mr. G said that the compression was very comfortable right from the beginning. He also was pleased that his legs didn't hurt so much at the end of the day. Mr. G put his feet up after his dog walks and used a recliner when he watched television. Mr. G's wound did heal eventually, but it took almost a year, and there were setbacks along the way. Mr. G said that the support of his wife, the fact that he was too old to get frustrated, and having a wound care team he trusted made all the difference in the world.

11

Arterial Wounds

*Dealing with Foot and Leg Wounds if
Your Circulation Is Poor*

*Mr. S is forty-seven years old, smokes, and has had diabetes since he
was a child. He has always taken his insulin as prescribed, but his diabetes is severe and he has developed foot wounds. His father, who also
suffered terribly from diabetes, had severe kidney failure and died of a
heart attack just three months before Mr. S's first meeting with us at
the clinic. Mr. S and his mother were devastated, not to mention scared
about what this would mean for Mr. S.*

*We examined his foot and saw a hard black wound on his big toe.
Mr. S was living at an assisted living center because he couldn't walk
on his foot. You could tell that for this very nice, bright man, coming to
see us was his last hope of finding a way to live on his own again.*

Many people with diabetes have poor circulation as well, also
called arterial disease. People may have arterial disease even without
diabetes. If you have an arterial ulcer* it means that you do not have
enough blood flowing *to* your legs and feet (venous ulcers are due to
impaired blood flow *from* your legs and feet back up to your heart).
These wounds are also called ischemic ulcers*. It is estimated that

between 5 to 20 percent of all leg ulcers are caused by problems with arteries.

Causes of Arterial Ulcers

Arteries carry blood leaving the heart to every part of the body. Arterial ulcers occur when arterial blood flow is interrupted, for example by narrowing of an artery. This can occur in any artery and can result from trauma or chronic disease (such as atherosclerosis, or hardening of the arteries, which is associated with smoking and unhealthy diet).

Warning Signs of Impaired Blood Flow to the Legs and Feet

Ischemia* means that there is not enough blood flowing to an organ or body part. In the case of arterial ulcers this usually means to the feet and legs. The feet and legs are usually the first places to be affected by hardening of the arteries. This artery hardening means that less blood is able to pass through the artery, which can result in ischemia in the area where blood was supposed to be flowing. It may then progress to

You are at higher risk for arterial ulcers if you:

- Are male
- Smoke
- Have diabetes mellitus
- Have hyperlipidemia or high cholesterol
- Have high blood pressure
- Are obese
- Are over sixty-five years old

The more risk factors you have, the higher at risk you are.

the hands. In many cases, no signs of impaired blood flow (or arterial disease) may be present until you find an ulcer on your leg or foot. The most common symptom of ischemia is pain, which can be severe and may progress from pain with walking or other activity to pain even while you are resting.

Pain in the calf or other leg muscles with walking or other exercise is similar to angina. Angina is when you have chest pain because the heart muscles are not receiving enough oxygen. Oxygen is essential for muscle functioning, and when a muscle does not have enough oxygen it hurts. This is because the vessels are too narrow to bring enough blood (which carries oxygen) to the muscles of the heart. In the heart muscle, this oxygen deficiency causes the pain of angina. In leg muscles, the same deficiency causes pain with exercise. This pain is often the first sign of arterial disease.

This leg pain, which can occur in any muscle that is fed by an artery that has narrowed, is pain that is noticed when you exercise (walking, for example). This pain goes away when you stop walking. It makes sense that the pain goes away if you stop walking if you think about why the pain is caused. The pain is caused by lack of oxygen, so if you stop walking then your muscle does not need as much oxygen and the pain goes away. You may have this pain in the calf, thigh, or buttocks. It can be measured by the distance you can walk before needing to stop to relieve the pain. Factors that tend to shorten the distance traveled before pain occurs include: obesity, smoking, and the extent of hardening of the arteries.

If you have this leg pain, you don't have to sit or adopt a particular position to relieve the discomfort: just rest and the pain will go away. But, as arterial disease gets worse, the distance shortens until, ultimately, you may feel pain even when resting.

Rest pain commonly occurs in the foot and can occur when you are asleep. This pain means that the blood cannot flow into the legs when you are lying down. Muscles always need oxygen or they will die, because they don't only need oxygen when you are active. Getting up and walking may provide some relief; however, it isn't the walking that is the key—lowering the leg to help the blood flow to the foot is the

Do You Have Poor Blood Flow (Arterial Insufficiency)?

- Do you have calf pain that worsens with exercise and is relieved by rest?
- Do you have calf pain while resting?
- Does getting up or hanging your foot and leg over the edge of the bed relieve the pain?
- Do you sometimes sleep in a chair because the pain in your legs hurts less that way?
- Do you have heart disease or diabetes, or have you ever had a stroke?

key to making this pain go away. Gravity helps blood flow into the foot and calf, which satisfies the muscle's need for oxygen and relieves the discomfort. By the time rest pain occurs, tissues in the foot are severely ischemic, whether or not an ulcer is present. Unless arterial flow is restored, an amputation may be the only choice to relieve pain, improve quality of life, and decrease the dangers associated with keeping dying tissues on the body (such as severe infection).

Where Do Arterial Ulcers Occur?

Arterial ulcers most commonly occur in the area around the toes (Figure 16). You may have black tips of the toes. Arterial ulcers are commonly found at the ends of arterial branches, especially at the tips of the toes, the corners of nail beds, or over bony prominences (the "knuckle" of the toes). Arterial ulcers can also occur on other areas of the foot and lower leg. The rest of the skin on your feet may be blue or red at times, and may be cool to the touch.

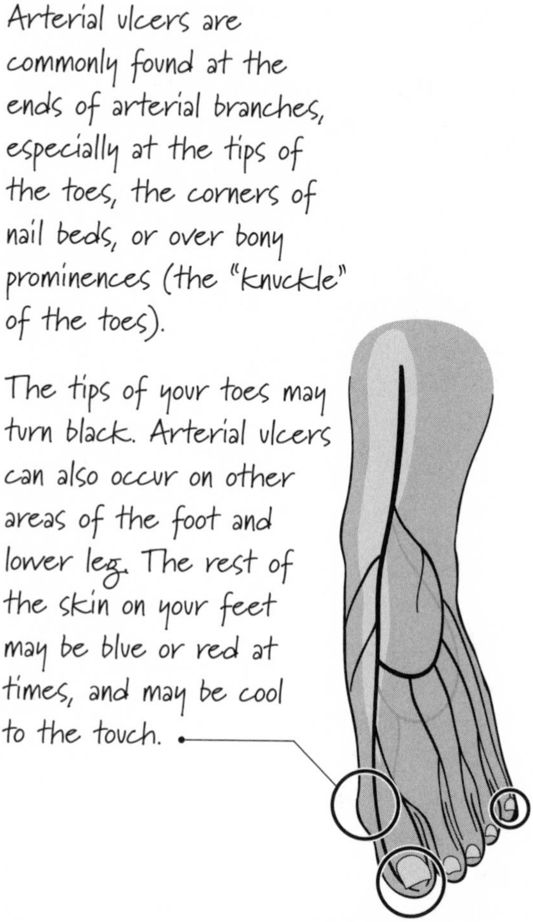

Arterial ulcers are commonly found at the ends of arterial branches, especially at the tips of the toes, the corners of nail beds, or over bony prominences (the "knuckle" of the toes).

The tips of your toes may turn black. Arterial ulcers can also occur on other areas of the foot and lower leg. The rest of the skin on your feet may be blue or red at times, and may be cool to the touch.

Figure 16: Arterial ulcers most commonly occur in the area around the toes.

Diagnostic Tests

Some things that your wound team may look for to determine whether you have arterial insufficiency may include:

- Pulses in the feet
- Seeing if your foot color pales when elevated and becomes deep red when dropped down (as the skin refills with blood)

- Cool, blue toes (which indicates that blood supply to the toes is severely decreased)

Your doctor may also order Doppler or other tests (described below) to see if you have arterial diseases.

Doppler Tests

A Doppler test measures blood flow in your legs. A cuff, like the one used to measure blood pressure in your arm, is used to measure the force of the blood flow. This cuff is wrapped around your arm and your blood pressure is measured. Then the leg on the same side of the body is then measured. The leg is usually measured in several places: the upper thigh, the lower thigh, the upper calf and the ankle. Arteries in the leg are usually more affected by arterial disease, so the pressure in the arm is then compared to the pressure in your leg. A lower blood pressure in your leg may mean that you have a narrowing in your leg arteries.

This test is quite easy to do and is not invasive (no needles). If you have diabetes, Doppler tests may show falsely high blood pressures because of hardening of the arteries. Therefore, if you have diabetes, other tests might be a better choice.

Toe Pressures

Toe pressures are measured in much the same way as in a Doppler test. A very small cuff is used to measure these pressures. Pressures in the toe should be about 70 percent of pressure in the arm. If the pressure is less than that, it indicates that there may be narrowing of the arteries. Toe pressures are a better choice for people with diabetes, as falsely high pressure readings are not found in the toe.

Transcutaneous Oxygen Levels

Transcutaneous oxygen levels are measured by sensors that measure oxygen that is being given off by the skin. This test can be particularly useful for diagnosing arterial disease in people who have very stiff vessels. The disadvantage is that oxygen can only be measured for very small areas.

Treatment of an Arterial Ulcer

The first goal in the treatment of an arterial ulcer is improving the blood flow to the legs and feet. Without blood flow, the ulcer won't heal. Options for improving blood flow include arterial bypass surgery or angioplasty (using a "balloon" to open up a blockage) and placement of stents (to keep the artery open and blood flowing). We talk more about surgical options for improving blood flow in Chapter 21. In addition, the ulcer must receive appropriate wound care. In general, medications are not effective when arterial disease has advanced to the point that ulcers are present.

Arterial bypass surgery may be the best way to restore arterial flow. The type and extent of bypass surgery depends on the ulcer's stage and location, as well as your general health. It is major surgery and so has risks associated with it, as with any surgery.

Less invasive interventions, such as angioplasty, are more commonly used for treatment of some types of arterial disease. Usually, a local (rather than a general) anesthetic is used during the procedure. General anesthesia is more dangerous to your health than local anesthetics. During angioplasty (also known as a "balloon" procedure), a catheter with a balloon is inserted into an artery in your groin. Using dye and watching on a monitor, the surgeon carefully maneuvers the catheter to the portion of the narrowed artery and then expands the balloon. The expanding balloon increases the diameter of the inside of the artery.

Stents are small metal structures that can be inserted into an artery after angioplasty to hold the artery open. They were developed to extend the amount of time that the artery remains open after angioplasty and reduce the need for surgery. Stent placement is gaining in popularity but the success rate of this procedure over time has yet to be determined. However, stents may be an alternative for those considered at too high a risk for arterial bypass surgery.

Taking Care of Your Feet if You Have Arterial Disease

Make sure that your feet are protected at all times. There are many types of protective footgear to choose from. Keep in mind that ischemic tissue can easily develop additional ulcers with little irritation or pressure. Even pressure from the foot resting on the bed or an ill-fitting protective boot can initiate new ulcers. Make sure your wound team carefully checks any protective devices you use for possible pressure points.

If the ulcer area contains dry necrotic tissue*, your wound team will probably continue to suggest a dry dressing. A dry necrotic toe (this can look mummified) will not cause further harm. However, these areas have no sensation and must be protected from injury. Ideally, this necrosis will demarcate (meaning the dying tissue will naturally separate from the living tissue). Once demarcation is complete, the digit will most likely fall off. If a loss of a toe seems imminent, it is important to talk to loved ones and your health-care professional about your feelings. It is important to be prepared.

If the arterial ulcer is wet or seems infected, it is important to consult your wound care professional. It may be important to remove the necrotic tissue* to protect you from further spread of infection. IV antibiotics may also be important. See Chapter 18 for the type of dressing to put on your arterial wound.

You can use these tips to help promote healing of your vascular ulcer and reduce your risk of developing new ulcers:

- Look at your skin every day. Use a moisturizer on dry, flaky skin but not on wounds (make sure that the moisturizer has been approved by your wound team—also see the section on "Dry Skin" in Chapter 35).
- Wear shoes that fit well, and always wear socks with shoes.
- Walking or other exercise in moderation can help (check with your wound team). Using your calf muscles can aid healing.
- Report any skin injury to your wound specialist.
- Don't smoke.
- Flex your feet up and down (as if you were using the gas pedal in a car) frequently when sitting.

Watch Out!

If you have arterial disease, especially if it is severe, elevating your legs and/or wearing compression stockings can make the blood flow to your feet *worse,* and can increase your pain. Talk to your health-care team if you are concerned about any of these issues.

- Elevate your legs whenever you sit (if you have venous disease).
- Wear your compression stockings as directed.
- Strive to maintain a target weight agreed upon by you and your health-care team.

We could see from the tests we had ordered that Mr. S had very poor blood flow in his legs. We suggested that he see a vascular surgeon, who felt that peripheral arterial bypass surgery would probably improve the blood flow, but not by much. Mr. S had the surgery, and his wound improved a little but never did heal completely.

When we asked Mr. S what his goal was, he said he wanted to be back at home. After discussion with Mr. S and his mother, we decided that although his wound was not likely to heal completely, we could keep his foot free of infection and keep him free of pain. We stressed the importance of quitting smoking in order to minimize worsening of his arterial disease. With his family, wound team, and home health services working together, we were able to get Mr. S back home. We still see him from time to time to make sure he is comfortable and ensure his wound isn't running his life.

12

Swelling

What Your Achy Feet Are Telling You

Have you wondered why your lower legs and feet at times seem to swell up like balloons? Have you wondered if there is something you can do for your loved one who complains of this swelling? As with so many other conditions, you don't have to "just deal with it." This chapter will teach you about this condition, also called edema, and what you can do to help you or your loved one.

Swelling in the lower legs can occur because of underlying medical problems (such as heart or kidney failure), venous disease, or lymphedema. Blockage of the venous system (or malfunctioning valves in the veins) causes blood and fluids to settle in the lower legs and feet, causing edema (venous ulcers were discussed in Chapter 10). In this chapter, we discuss how to control swelling caused by venous disease (edema) or lymphedema.

Lymphedema

Lymphatic vessels, unlike blood vessels, do not transport blood. Instead, the lymphatic vessels remove waste products and excess fluids from the skin and then transport them to large veins. Blockage of the lymphatic system can lead to lymphedema.

Lymphedema is not the same thing as edema from venous insufficiency. However, untreated venous insufficiency can progress to edema, which is treated the same way as lymphedema.

Why does it occur? Lymphedema may be inherited: some people are born with lymphatics that are not formed properly. It is often caused by injury to the lymphatic vessels (such as surgery after cancer treatment or other trauma). The exact cause of inherited lymphedema is unknown. It usually occurs due to poorly developed or missing lymph nodes. You may have had lymphedema since birth or it might not have developed until later in life.

Symptoms of lymphedema include severe fatigue, a heavy swollen leg, discoloration of the skin in the area of lymphedema, changes to the skin, and eventually deformity (known as elephantiasis*). Lymphedema can occur in both legs or only in one. Lymphedema affects both men and women.

Treating Lymphedema

Methods to control edema and lymphedema are often similar. They include elevation of the affected limb, compression therapy, and, sometimes, medication or surgery.

Medications

Medications to reduce swelling in the legs are not often the best treatment. Diuretics (water pills) do not address the underlying problem of venous disease or lymphedema, and can cause dehydration. You may, however, need to take diuretics for other conditions, such as heart failure or high blood pressure.

Elevating Your Legs

An effective method of reducing edema is to elevate the leg and allow gravity to drain fluid from it. This is best accomplished if your legs are elevated above the level of the heart. This can be done in a recliner chair with the feet up high, for example. Unfortunately, this position may be very uncomfortable (that is, may make you short of breath) if you have a heart or lung condition. In this case, any elevation that you can tolerate is beneficial.

Compression Bandaging

The best way to control swelling, heal venous ulcers, and prevent future ulcers is to use compression therapy (either compression wrapping or stockings) (Figure 17). Various rigid and flexible types of compression bandages are available. However, before you start compression therapy, your wound care team will ensure that you have enough blood flow to your feet so your circulation will not be cut off, as this may cause further damage to your tissues. Your wound specialist may do this by checking for a pulse, and may order other tests also, such as arterial blood flow tests (described in Chapter 11). Your wound specialist will then decide how many layers of compression bandaging are right for you. You may need as little as one layer, or as many as four layers.

Usually, when you have a venous leg ulcer, compression bandaging should be used at least two weeks after you have completely healed. If the compression bandaging is stopped too early, you may get another ulcer because the skin has not regained its strength. After you completely heal, keep wearing the compression bandaging for two more weeks, then start wearing compression stockings. Compression stockings are something you'll need to wear for the rest of your life in order to reduce the chance of getting another ulcer.

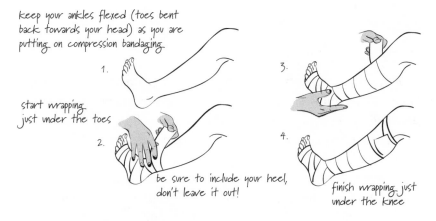

Figure 17: Managing leg swelling and edema.

A Warning About Compression

It is very important that your wound team assess you to make sure you do not have arterial disease (poor blood flow from your heart to your legs) or unstable heart failure before using compression bandaging or compression stockings.

Compression Pumps

Pumps to control lymphedema provide compression and are often covered by Medicare and most insurance companies. These devices typically work through the use of a pneumatic sleeve that gently moves the lymph fluid. You may often receive treatment on a pump for 10–15 minutes before a session of manual lymphatic drainage, or use the pump for an hour or so a day. Some people benefit from home use of sequential pumps, which are made by several manufacturers. Many people find these pumps very comfortable and some even fall asleep while using them.

Compression Stockings

Once your venous leg ulcer has healed, or if you have lymphedema, it is very likely you will then need lifelong use of compression stockings. This will reduce your chances of developing more leg ulcers in the future. Stockings are available in several classes of tightness, measured at the ankle. The tighter the stockings are, the more effective they can be, but also the more uncomfortable they can become. Any strength that you can tolerate is usually better than nothing at all—check with your wound team. It is important that you go to a knowledgeable fitter who can measure you

Table 3: Different Types of Compression Stockings

Strength (tightness)	Use
>60 mmHg	Elephantiasis, irreversible lymphedema
40–50 mmHg	Previous, recurrent venous ulcers
30–40 mmHg	Moderate edema, severe varicose veins, previous venous ulcers
20–30 mmHg	Varicose veins, mild edema
16–20 mmHg (dress support stockings)	When tighter stockings are not tolerated. These stockings also come in many colors (not just brown), so they can be a more physically attractive option to wear.
8–13 mmHg (thromboembolic stockings or other light stockings)	When tighter stockings are not tolerated or when edema and arterial disease are both present

properly so your stockings fit well and are comfortable. Generally, you should go to your fitter early in the day, before your swelling builds up. Different types of compression stockings are shown in Table 3.

Stockings only need to be knee-high to be effective. Once they are higher than that (i.e., thigh-high or pantyhose length), they can be very difficult to put on and very uncomfortable. However, if you prefer the higher lengths, they work just fine. Stockings can often also be available custom-made (great for people with hard-to-fit legs and feet), which do not cover the toes (can be more comfortable if you have foot deformities, but the downside is that you may need to wear another sock on top) or with a zipper (can make the stockings much easier to put on). Be wary of using a stocking with a zipper if you have diabetic neuropathy (poor sensation in your legs due to diabetes): you run the risk of zipping up your skin and not noticing it.

Stockings also vary quite a bit in cost (from $20 per pair to $200). Insurance often covers stockings (for more information, see Chapter 39). Generally, the looser the stockings, the less expensive they are. If insurance does not cover your stockings, one trick is to wear two pairs of lighter stockings at the same time, instead of one tight pair. This method can also make your stockings much easier to put on. Make sure you talk to your wound team before making any changes to the prescription you were given. Tips to help you keep wearing your stockings are shown in Table 4.

Table 4: Tricks to Help You Stick to Wearing Your Stockings

Problem	Solution
Arthritis in hands or back, making it difficult to bend over and pull on stockings	• Use rubber gloves • Devices are available to pull on stockings
Cost	• Check with different manufacturers • Seek out different strengths and styles and compare cost (e.g., with/without toes, with/without zipper)
Comfort	• Seek out different strengths and styles and compare feel (e.g., with/without toes, with/without zipper) • Try different lengths (e.g., knee high, thigh high)
Cosmetic appearance	• Wear another sock or fashion stockings on top of compression stocking • Choose different lengths of stockings • Choose different materials (e.g., cotton, nylon) • Select different colors

Lymphatic Massage

Manual lymph drainage is done by a trained professional and consists of gentle, rhythmic massaging of the skin to stimulate the flow of lymph and its return to the blood circulation system. The treatment is very comfortable and nonaggressive. A typical session lasts approximately forty to sixty minutes, depending on the severity and extent of the lymphedema. This treatment can be quite costly and can require a serious time commitment on your part. However, lymphatic drainage is often covered by private insurance companies and by Medicare and can be effective in reducing swelling.

Table 4: (*continued*)

Problem	Solution
Forget to put on stockings	• Put on before getting out of bed in the morning
Care	• Use gloves to apply • Wash on "delicate" setting in the washing machine (or hand wash), hang to dry
Replacement	• Replace stockings every 3–6 months (otherwise elastic goes and the stockings are no longer as effective)
Itching	• Try a different material of stocking (e.g., cotton vs. nylon) • Try a special anti-itch cream (as recommended by your wound team), but avoid use of creams at the same time you wear your stocking because creams can destroy the elastic (suggestion: wear stockings in daytime and cream at night)
Can't figure out how to put stockings on	• Go back to your stocking fitter (or find another one) and ask for a review of technique

Exercise

Exercise is a very important part of controlling edema. Walking, in particular, helps blood flow back up to the heart from the legs and feet. Even ten to fifteen minutes of walking a day can be beneficial.

Pool therapy combined with manual lymphatic drainage can help people with lymphedema.

Weight Control

The rates of lymphedema in people who are morbidly obese are very high. Reducing weight may help your lymphedema symptoms. It is important to maintain a healthy weight. Diet and exercise regimes should be discussed with trained health-care professionals.

Surgery

Surgical techniques for correcting lymphedema may help some people when areas of lymphedema can be surgically removed. Other times, the lymph vessels themselves can be operated on. But, be aware that surgical wounds on legs that swell easily are often slow to heal. If your legs swell easily and you have to have a procedure on your legs, it is a good idea to have a plan in place with your surgeon about how to manage swelling before you have the procedure. The tightness of the compression will not make your wound heal more slowly, and may actually allow for quicker healing.

Skin Care

People with lymphedema or those who have had lymph nodes removed are at a higher risk for infections of the affected areas. A specific regimen of thorough but gentle cleansing followed by moisturizing will help keep the skin in the best health possible. Educating yourself about the signs and symptoms of infections is also important, since awareness is the key to early identification and treatment. Untreated infections can further damage an already impaired lymphatic system and lead to more severe lymphedema and skin ulcers.

PART FIVE

Acute Wounds

If acute wounds persist for several weeks with little or no improvement, they are known as chronic wounds. Chronic wounds are much more difficult to heal than acute wounds.

Acute wounds can occur in two ways: intentionally during surgery or accidentally by trauma. Surgery produces a controlled acute wound, which means that the incision is intentionally made, but in a way to minimize unwanted effects such as infection. Traumatic wounds (for example, burns) can range from simple to severe.

In this section, we discuss different types of acute wounds and how you can most effectively deal with them so that they heal well and don't become chronic.

13
Healing After Surgery

A surgical wound is an intentional break in the skin as a result of surgery; these breaks in the skin are called incisions and are created by some sort of surgical tool, like a scalpel. In a healthy person, this type of wound responds well to postoperative care and heals without any major problems in a relatively short period of time.

Sometimes wounds made during surgery can take a long time to heal and become chronic. Healing depends on the type of wound you have, and if you have any underlying medical conditions that contribute to poor wound healing. In this chapter, we'll look at how to promote optimal healing of the wounds you or your loved one has from surgery.

Factors that Affect Healing

Several factors can greatly affect the course of wound healing after surgery.

AGE

Infants: In premature infants and infants up to age 1, the immune system and other body systems aren't fully developed, so there's a greater risk for infection before, during, and after surgery. Keeping tools sterile (cleansed of any bacteria) is key for everyone who undergoes surgery, and particularly for very young people.

Older adults (over the age of sixty years): Skin becomes thinner and less elastic with age. The cells that repair tissues and fight infection reduce in number, and the blood flow to the skin is not as strong as it used to be. As a result, surgical wounds in older adults heal more slowly, increasing the risk of infection.

ILLNESS

In most cases, an illness that you had before your operation delays or complicates healing after surgery. Unfortunately, it isn't always possible to delay surgery while another problem resolves itself. In these cases, the care plan must include measures that minimize the impact of the preexisting condition on the healing process. Here are some conditions that require consideration when surgery is indicated.

- *Diabetes mellitus*: Diabetes slows healing in many ways and increases your risk of infection. Diabetic neuropathy (inflammation and degeneration of peripheral nerves), if present, may interfere with the normal function of blood vessels, and may result in decreased blood flow to the surgical incision site.
- *Medications*: Drugs, including steroids and chemotherapy agents, may reduce the ability of your immune system to function at its best. Therefore, if you are taking these medications, wound healing may be delayed, and risk of infection can be high. If you think your wound is not healing due to your medications, talk to your doctor *before* stopping any medications.
- *Cancer*: Either treatment for cancer, or the cancer itself, can affect your body's ability to heal (see Chapter 30). Also, cancer treatment may require aggressive pain management while you are recovering from surgery. Often a care plan is needed that manages such symptoms as nausea and vomiting, which may be worse after surgery. Medications for all these problems can affect your appetite and nutrition, and may lead to further problems with wound healing.
- *Blood circulation*: Disorders that impair blood flow, such as coronary artery disease, peripheral vascular disease (see

Part IV), and hypertension can cause problems by reducing the flow of blood reaching the incision site. If you have one of these conditions, you need to discuss this with your doctor. In order to have an optimal outcome in surgery, you need a care plan that includes interventions to improve circulation.

- *Severe lung disease*: During healing, white blood cells need oxygen to produce the substances they use to kill bacteria (and other infectious agents) and also need oxygen to repair the wound itself. Therefore, adequate oxygen is critical to the healing process. Any condition that reduces overall oxygenation or the amount of oxygen reaching the wound slows the healing process.

NUTRITION

Proper nutrition plays an important role in how well you will heal after surgery. See Chapter 32 for more information.

INFECTION

Infection can also delay or impair healing. See Chapter 15 for more information.

How Your Surgeon Closes a Wound

Your surgeon determines the appropriate method of wound closure based on the wound's severity; in most cases, sutures (also called stitches) are used. In suturing, a natural or synthetic thread is used to stitch the wound closed. Sutures typically remain in place for seven to ten days, depending on the wound's severity, the type of tissue involved, and whether healing is progressing as expected. The surgeon may choose to use skin staples or clips as an alternative to sutures if cosmetic results aren't an issue (staples and clips can leave more visible scars than sutures). These closures secure a wound faster than sutures and, because they're made of surgical stainless steel, tissue reaction is minimal. Properly placed staples and clips distribute tension

Why Sutures (Stitches) or Staples Can't Be Used to Heal Your Chronic Wound

Unfortunately, sutures or staples work to heal only acute wounds, not chronic wounds. Once a wound has become chronic, simply closing up the outside layer of skin will not allow the deep layers to heal. The sutures or staples will ultimately just pop open, or worse, you may develop a deep infection. For a chronic wound (that is, a wound that's been open for a long time), you need to allow it to heal from the inside out.

evenly along the suture line, reducing tissue trauma and compression and promoting healing.

Smaller wounds with little drainage can be closed with adhesive skin closures, such as Steri-Strips or butterfly closures. As with staples and clips, these closures cause little tissue reaction. Adhesive closures can be used after suture or staple removal to provide ongoing support for a healing incision.

Caring for Your Wound After Surgery

After surgery, guidelines for proper care of your wound vary depending on several factors, so make sure you follow your surgeon's instructions. You may want to ask for written instructions to help you remember the details at home. Focus on keeping the wound clean and protecting it from accidental injury like bumping or scratching. In this section, we provide basic information about post-surgery wound care.

Wound Dressings

The incision dressing shields the wound against bacteria (and other infectious agents) and protects the skin surface from wound drainage that can irritate it. The dressing for your immediate postoperative wound care will be chosen while you are in the hospital.

Your nurse will use sterile supplies when dressing the wound in order to prevent infection, and will change the dressing as often as needed to absorb drainage and keep the surrounding skin dry. Keeping the wound exposed to air without a dressing may dry it out too much; wound dressings help prevent this from happening.

 Before you leave the hospital after surgery, make sure you understand:

- *Signs and symptoms of wound infection*: These include increased tenderness, deep or increased pain at the wound site, and fever or swelling (especially if it occurs between postoperative days three and five). Report these to your health-care team immediately.
- *How to take an accurate temperature reading*: You may want to buy a new thermometer so you can do this. Although digital ones are more expensive, they are very easy to read.
- *Proper wound care*: This concerns keeping the incision clean and dry, including methods used to clean the wound; proper hand-washing technique; and necessary supplies, including where to get them.
- *Wound dressings*: Determine the type, how to apply them, and where to obtain them.
- *What you are allowed to do*: Consult with your health-care team about the types and levels of permissible activity, such as restrictions on lifting (if applicable), driving, when you may shower or bathe, and when you can expect to return to work.
- *Follow-up appointments*: Make sure you know when you need to see your health-care team again.

Learning About Your Wound

You are the most important part of the care plan, particularly after a surgery. By the time of hospital discharge, you (or your caregiver) should understand and/or be able to perform proper wound care. You'll be taught about how to keep the wound clean, how to have proper hand-washing technique, and how to apply the dressing.

After surgery, you and/or your caregiver need to know the ways that you can promote healing and prevent infection. Make sure that your health-care team has talked to you about this and has instructed you sufficiently. Ask them to write down any important points you may want to remember later. If you don't understand or don't think you'll be able to do it, speak up and tell them your concerns.

Why Isn't My Wound Healing After Surgery?

Most surgical wounds heal without any problems. However, some complications that might arise include infection, excessive bleeding, and dehiscence* (when the wound spontaneously splits open).

Infection

Wound infection is the most common wound complication as well as the second most common health-care–associated infection. Preventing wound infection requires meticulous attention to sterile technique when caring for an acute wound.

If your doctor thinks you may have an infection in your surgical wound, he/she may do the following:

- Obtain a wound culture and sensitivity test
- Administer antibiotics
- Irrigate (wash out) the wound
- Open up the wound, then dress the wound and loosely pack it, if necessary
- Monitor wound drainage

Bleeding

An excessive amount of bleeding may sometimes occur from the wound as a result of damage to blood vessels. If this happens and you lose a lot of blood, your medical team may need to administer intravenous fluids, or even a blood transfusion, to increase blood pressure. Meanwhile, they will determine the source of bleeding. Place pressure using your hand on the site of the bleeding and notify your doctor or wound team immediately.

Dehiscence

Dehiscence refers to a wound that appears to have healed, but then breaks open. This is most likely to occur when the scar tissue is not able to hold the incision closed without sutures. The first sign of dehiscence may be an abscess or a gush of fluid from the wound, or you may feel a "popping" sensation after sneezing, coughing, or vomiting. Dehiscence can occur after any type of surgery, but abdominal wounds are more likely to dehisce than chest wounds. Some patients who have mesh placed in their abdominal wounds may experience dehiscence.

To prevent wound dehiscence, learn how to support the incision with a pillow or cushion before you change position, cough, or sneeze. Speak to your health-care team about this before you leave the hospital, if you can.

If a wound is not improving a month or so after surgery, or if the wound reopens (dehiscence), call your surgeon. Your surgical wound may now be a chronic wound, and you may need to see a chronic wound specialist.

14

Traumatic Wounds

Burns, Cuts, and More

Mr. P is a gentleman with a particularly troublesome traumatic wound. When he was thirteen years old, he was in a hunting accident, and fragments of gunshot were sprayed into his left calf. Mr. P says that he was taken to the doctor and most of the fragments were removed from his calf. It was clear, though, nearly sixty years later, that there was still gunshot residue in his leg, because his wound would not heal.

A traumatic wound is a sudden, unplanned injury to the skin that can range from minor (such as a skinned knee) to severe (such as a gunshot wound). Sometimes a traumatic wound can cause as many long-term problems as a chronic wound.

If you or your loved one suffers a traumatic wound, call an ambulance. If the wound is severe, if there is a lot of bleeding, or if the wound is deep, you may need to go to the emergency room at the nearest hospital. Time is critical, especially if your injury is severe.

The medical team will first make sure that your breathing and circulation are normal. Although focusing first on the injury itself may seem natural, an open airway and pumping heart take priority. Only then can care of the wound itself take place.

In this chapter, we discuss how to treat minor skin injuries and wounds. If you have a skin injury from trauma, however, you need to call your doctor or go to the nearest emergency room.

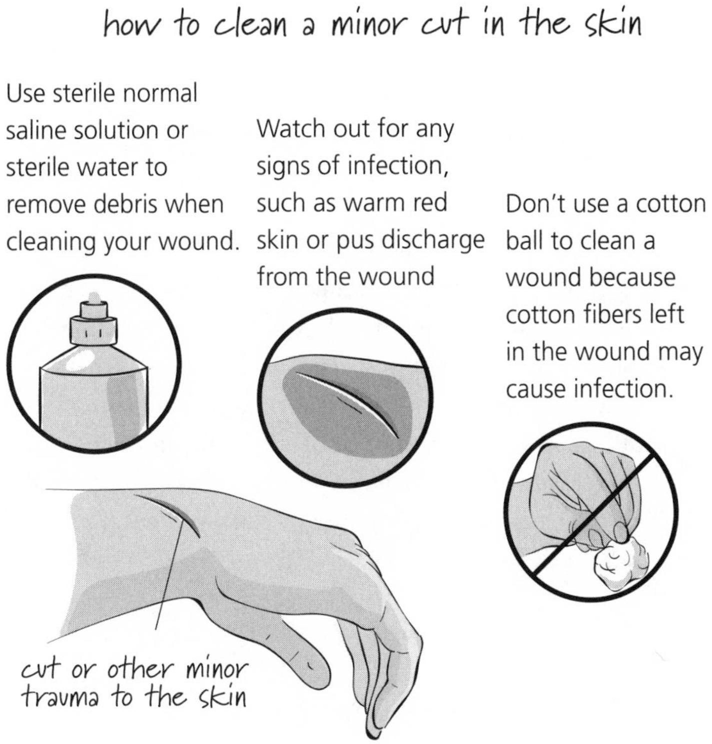

how to clean a minor cut in the skin

Use sterile normal saline solution or sterile water to remove debris when cleaning your wound.

Watch out for any signs of infection, such as warm red skin or pus discharge from the wound

Don't use a cotton ball to clean a wound because cotton fibers left in the wound may cause infection.

cut or other minor trauma to the skin

Figure 18: How to clean a minor cut in the skin.

There are many types of minor skin injuries, including abrasions, lacerations, skin tears, and bites. Figure 18 illustrates proper care of minor cuts.

Abrasions

An abrasion occurs when a mechanical force, such as friction or shearing, scrapes away a partial thickness of the skin. Unless an unusually large amount of skin is involved or an infection develops, an abrasion is one of the least complicated traumatic wounds to treat.

- Flush the area of the abrasion with normal saline solution or wound cleaning solution.
- Use a sterile 4-by-4-inch gauze pad moistened with normal saline solution to remove dirt or gravel and gently rub toward the entry point to work contaminants back out the way they entered.
- If the wound is extremely dirty, it may need to be scrubbed with a surgical brush. Scrubbing a wound should be done only by a health-care professional. As this can be a painful process, it should be done as gently as possible.
- Allow a small wound to dry and form a scab. For small wounds, apply a small amount of antibiotic ointment and cover with a dressing. Cover larger wounds with a nonadherent pad or petroleum gauze, apply antibacterial ointment if ordered, and a light dressing.

Lacerations

A laceration is a tear in the skin caused by a sharp object, such as metal, glass, or wood. It can also be caused by trauma that produces high shearing force. A laceration has jagged, irregular edges and its severity depends on its cause, size, depth, and location.

Skin Tears

A skin tear is a specific type of laceration or abrasion that most often affects older adults (sixty years and older). As skin ages, it becomes thinner, drier, and less elastic, and so it is more fragile overall. Although skin tears can occur anywhere on the body, 80 percent of them occur on the hands or arms. The next most common location is the lower legs.

In a skin tear, friction alone—or shearing force plus friction—separates layers of skin. This type of injury may be, but is not always, preventable through careful handling of the individual (for example, during transferring from bed to chair).

Most Common Causes of Skin Tears

1. Wheelchair injuries (25 percent)
2. Impact with objects (e.g., furniture, wheelchairs, bed rails, lifts, tub chairs) (25 percent)
3. Transfers (18 percent)
4. Falls (12 percent)
5. Removal of tape or other adhesives

 Preventing Skin Tears

As people get older, especially over the age of sixty-five years, their skin becomes more prone to tearing. You can help prevent skin tears by:

- Learning to properly lift and transfer the person
- Placing padding on surfaces such as bed rails, as well as arm rests and foot supports on wheelchairs
- Using nonstick dressings or paper tape
- Removing tape carefully
- Speaking up if dressing removal is painful
- Applying a moisturizer twice a day

Older adults who are dependent for their activities of daily living (i.e., dressing, bathing, positioning, and transferring) are at the highest risk for skin tears. Those who are independent and ambulatory have the second highest risk, with injuries due to transfers to and from wheelchairs and tub chairs. Visual impairment can also increase the risk of bumping into objects.

Bites

When assessing a bite wound, it's important to quickly discover the bite's source. This helps the health-care team determine which bacteria or toxins may be present and the likely type of wound. For example, a human bite can cause a puncture wound. The human mouth is full of bacteria, and these puncture wounds can result in these bacteria entering the skin and causing potentially life-threatening infections. A bite from a dog, cat, or rodent can introduce deadly infectious diseases, such as rabies, into a wound. A dog can generate a lot of pressure when biting and cause a crushing-type wound. Cat bites cause relatively little tissue damage but can introduce dangerous infections into the deep tissues.

Call your doctor or go to the nearest emergency room if you have suffered a bite. You may need intravenous antibiotics or a tetanus vaccine.

Burns

A burn is an acute wound caused by exposure to extreme heat or extreme cold, electricity, caustic chemicals, or radiation. The degree of tissue damage caused by a burn depends on the source and the duration of exposure. Care for a burn depends on the type and severity of the burn, your general health before the injury, and whether another injury (for example, lung injury from smoke inhalation) was sustained at the same time as the burn. The goals of burn treatment are:

1. To reduce pain
2. To remove dirt and dead tissue
3. To use a wound dressing that helps healing.

Sometimes skin grafts are used to help heal burns (see Chapter 21).

Your health-care practitioner will determine the size of the burn. Usually, burn size is expressed as a percentage of total body surface

area. The larger the burn, the more serious the injury is. The traditional method of assessing burn severity was by depth: first degree,
second degree, and third degree.

*We explained to Mr. P that his wound was not likely to heal as long as
the gunshot residue remained in his leg. He agreed to let us try to take
the foreign material out in the clinic. We knew this would be very difficult as the back of his leg was heavily scarred. We used a needle to freeze
the skin in the area, and with a scalpel we were able to remove the
pieces of shot from his leg. Immediately after this procedure, the wound
was larger than when he came in because we had to remove the material that was keeping the wound from healing. Mr. P was upset at first,
but we explained to him that this larger, clean wound had a better
chance of healing than the smaller wound that had a foreign body in
it. Mr. P also showed signs of venous disease, so we sent him home with
compression bandaging. Six months later Mr. P's wound had healed.*

PART SIX

Nonhealing Wounds

When all standard approaches to healing a chronic wound fail, the wound is classified as nonhealing. Nonhealing wounds can be a very distressing problem for you and your loved ones, and frustrating for your health-care professional, who wants to be able to help you heal.

There are medical and nonmedical reasons why a wound may not heal. In this section, the most common reasons wounds fail to heal will be discussed.

15
Infected Wounds

You've properly tended to your wound but it is not healing. In fact, it is looking worse as time goes on. Now what?

If your wound is not healing, you and your wound team need to make sure that it is not infected. All wounds that have been open for a few days have bacteria growing in them. This is normal and does not mean that the wound is infected. An infected wound means that the wound has so much bacteria that normal wound healing is prevented.

Studies suggest that infection may be the cause of almost half of all nonhealing wounds. Some chronic diseases (such as diabetes) can increase your risk of developing infections in an open wound. If an infection remains undetected, the wound won't heal. Therefore, you can help your wound team by being vigilant for any signs of infection that may occur.

Figure 19 shows signs of infection that you should watch out for, and Figure 20 shows signs of infection that your wound team may look for.

Bone Infection

Another word for bone infection is osteomyelitis*. Osteomyelitis is a serious complication in which bacteria are growing in the bone.

If your wound team suspects a deep infection in the wound, they may need to make sure that the infection does not reach all the way to the bone. They may be particularly concerned about bone infection if your wound is deep and goes all the way down to the bone.

Some signs of infection that **you** should watch out for:

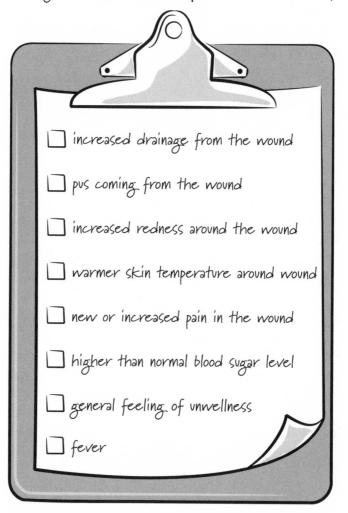

- ☐ increased drainage from the wound
- ☐ pus coming from the wound
- ☐ increased redness around the wound
- ☐ warmer skin temperature around wound
- ☐ new or increased pain in the wound
- ☐ higher than normal blood sugar level
- ☐ general feeling of unwellness
- ☐ fever

Figure 19: Signs of infection that you should watch out for.

Some signs of infection that **your wound team** may look for:

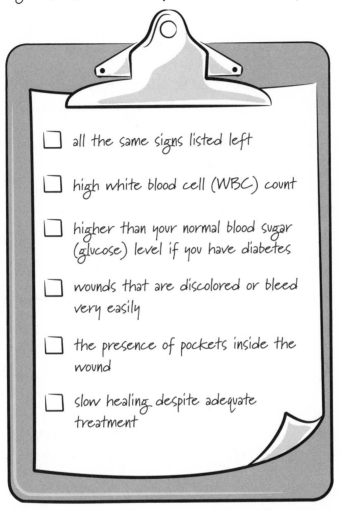

- all the same signs listed left
- high white blood cell (WBC) count
- higher than your normal blood sugar (glucose) level if you have diabetes
- wounds that are discolored or bleed very easily
- the presence of pockets inside the wound
- slow healing despite adequate treatment

Figure 20: Signs of infection that your wound team may look for.

Some tests that your team may order to see if you have a bone infection include:

- An X-ray of the affected area (but it can take weeks before any changes can be seen on an X-ray)
- Magnetic resonance imaging (MRI) or computerized tomography (CT or CAT) scan (these are the best painless, non-invasive tests)
- A bone biopsy (not as often done because it is invasive, but it is probably the best test to diagnose bone infection)

Treatment of Infected Wounds

Depending on how deep your wound infection is, your wound team may treat you with one or more of the following:

- Liquids, creams, or wound dressings that have antibacterial treatments in them (see Chapter 18)
- Antibiotics that you take by mouth
- Intravenous antibiotics

Usually, intravenous antibiotics are given only if you have a very deep infection and especially if you have infection of the bone. If the bone is not infected, you may need only a couple of weeks of intravenous antibiotics. However, if the bone is infected, you may need several weeks' worth. Often, these antibiotics can be given to you at home so you don't always need to be admitted to the hospital to receive them. If the infection has spread into the rest of your body, you may also be given intravenous medication.

16
Unusual Wounds

Ms. R is a twenty-nine-year-old woman who works as a consultant out of her home. She has struggled with Crohn's disease for ten years. One day she developed what she described as a "purple pimple" on her leg. It was too painful to even touch.

She went to bed that night and when she woke up, the area on her leg was very painful and had grown in size dramatically. She went to the emergency room, where she was given some ointment for the wound. However, after several days, the wound continued to increase in size and become even more painful.

If your wound takes a really long time to heal, your wound team may do a skin biopsy to see if the cause of your wound is one of the conditions described in this chapter.

Unusual wounds can take a long time for health-care teams to diagnose properly. Sometimes, your wound team can tell what the cause of the wound is simply by looking at it; other times, the only way to determine the cause of the wound is to do a skin biopsy* (see Chapter 4).

Pyoderma Gangrenosum

Pyoderma gangrenosum (also known as PG) causes ulcers to form, usually on the lower legs, but it can occur anywhere. Another common area for PG to occur is around stomas (see Chapter 27). Ulcers usually start out looking like a small bug bite or a blood blister but they may grow rapidly for some time until they are quite large. They are often very painful, and have raised, purplish-blue irregular borders. A substance that looks like pus may drain from little holes around the wound.

About half of people with PG ulcers have an underlying disease (usually Crohn's disease, ulcerative colitis, rheumatoid arthritis, non-Hodgkin's lymphoma, or multiple myeloma). The other half of people with PG ulcers don't have any other disease.

Not a lot is known about PG ulcers, but they are thought to be due to an immune system problem. If your wound team suspects you have PG, they may do a skin biopsy. Unfortunately, a skin biopsy only helps to diagnose PG about half of the time. The reason to do the skin biopsy is to make sure that the wound is not caused by something else.

Pyoderma gangrenosum can be tricky to treat. Treatments are usually directed at the immune system and at reducing the amount of inflammation in and around the wound. Your wound team may inject a steroid into the wound or give you steroids or immune-suppressing drugs to take by mouth or through an intravenous.

One unusual thing about PG wounds is that if they are surgically debrided, they can become a lot larger very quickly. In fact, among those people who are prone to developing PG wounds, any trauma (such as banging your shin against a chair) can result in a PG ulcer. Some wounds (but not most) that are slow to heal after surgery may be due to PG. Once you know you are prone to developing a PG wound, see your wound team within a few days so you can begin treatment while the ulcer is still small and can be healed quickly.

Hidradenitis Suppurativa

Hidradenitis suppurativa is a chronic inflammation in the underarms, groin, and around the anus. In this disease, painful lumps in the skin form and can fill with pus. Skin has many functions, and one of them is to help you sweat and cool off so you don't overheat. Sweat glands are found in the skin, and are more frequently present in certain parts of the body, such as the palms and soles. One type of sweat gland opens into hair follicles and is found in areas where hair typically grows, such as the scalp, groin, and underarms. Problems with these glands can lead to hidradenitis suppurativa.

Usually, hidradenitis suppurativa can be treated by injections of steroids into the lumps, but you may need treatment with medications by mouth also. Antibiotics may be used to control infection. In the case of severe, extensive HS, a plastic surgeon may surgically remove the sweat glands in the affected area.

Necrobiosis Lipoidica Diabeticorum

Necrobiosis Lipoidica Diabeticorum (NLD) causes ulcers, usually in people with diabetes. It occurs in 3 percent of people with diabetes, and 90 percent of the time in women. Unlike the foot ulcers that occur in some people with diabetes (discussed in Chapter 8), NLD is not due to nerve damage (neuropathy) or poor blood circulation and is not related to how well sugars are controlled.

NLD ulcers, which may be very painful, typically occur on the shins (as opposed to the more common foot ulcers) and may occur on both legs. They may start out as an area of skin discoloration, and an injury can cause the discolored area to ulcerate. It is not known why some people develop NLD and others don't.

Your wound team may do a skin biopsy to help diagnose NLD. Treatment is often with injections of steroid into the wound to reduce the inflammation.

Other Causes

There are many other unusual causes of ulcers (such as vasculitis and Behcet's disease). All of these are usually diagnosed with skin biopsies. Many can be treated, so be sure to speak to your wound specialist.

When Ms. R first came to our clinic, it had been several weeks since she first noticed the bump on her leg and her situation had become much worse. Even after several more trips to the emergency room, she was in a lot of pain and looking for answers.

When we first saw her, we felt that she had a PG ulcer, given its deep purple color and unusual border. The history of Crohn's disease also pointed toward PG. We injected steroids into her wound, which was painful for Ms. R, but we explained that this would help her heal more quickly and would help with her pain in the long run. We also started Ms. R on an oral antibiotic to treat an infection that had crept into the wound over the previous weeks.

Two weeks later, the steroid injections had worked well and her pain had improved; after three more months, her wound was healed and she was without any pain.

We told Ms. R that since she has PG, she may develop ulcers from time to time, but the most important thing was to call us or another wound clinic or dermatologist right away while the ulcers were small and more likely to heal quickly with the right treatment.

17
Still Not Healing . . .
What Are We Missing?

Some issues that may slow or prevent healing can be quite easily diagnosed with the help of your wound care team. We will discuss these issues in this chapter.

Cancer in the Wound

If your wound is very slow to heal, your wound team may do a skin biopsy (see Chapter 4). One reason to do a skin biopsy is to make sure there is no cancer in the wound. Often, a cancer in the wound is quite easily treated, once it is diagnosed, by having it removed.

Medications

Many commonly used medications (over-the-counter and prescription) may slow or prevent wound healing. Types of medications that may slow wound healing are shown in Figure 21 (page 139).

Always tell your medical team about all the medications you are taking, including over-the-counter and prescription drugs.

When Your Treatment Plan Is Hard to Follow

Sometimes nonmedical factors affect the healing process, and you need to discuss them with your wound team. Financial, cultural, or

Some Signs of Cancer in the Wound

- The wound grows rapidly (over a few weeks) or is growing above skin level
- The wound may bleed easily
- The skin around the wound may be very itchy
- The wound may drain a lot
- The wound may have a foul odor
- Wound care professionals say your wound does not look typical

Many wounds that do not have cancer have many of the same signs. The only way to know for sure is to have a skin biopsy. Often, your wound team may decide not to biopsy the wound right away, but to wait and see if it improves with treatment.

caregiving considerations may be getting in the way of following a recommended treatment plan for yourself or a loved one. Your wound team may not fully appreciate their importance to you unless you bring up the subject.

Money Issues

Whether or not you can afford the recommended treatment will affect your ability to follow through on your team's treatment plan. You need to let your wound team know this if it is the case. The team should do their best to help you and may take one or more of the following steps:

- Consult social services to determine if alternative payment sources can be found.

Types of medications that may slow wound healing
or increase your risk of wound infection:

- Nonsteroidal anti-inflammatories (for example, naproxen, and ibuprofen)
- Steroids (for example, prednisone)
- Some blood pressure and heart medications (for example, calcium channel blockers, which may cause ankle swelling)
- Antivirals
- Antibiotics
- Anti-cancer agents (that is, chemotherapy)
- Some herbal medications (for example, goldenseal may increase leg swelling, aloe vera can cause skin irritation if used frequently in people with wounds)

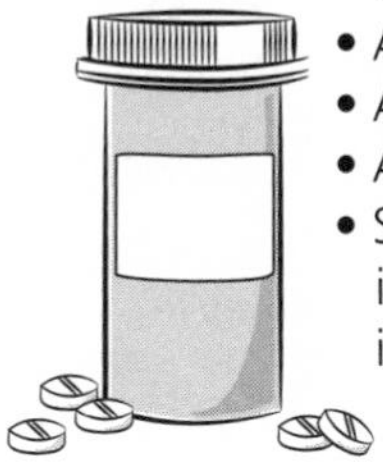

Figure 21: Types of medications that may slow wound healing.

- Make changes to the treatment plan in order to decrease your costs. Cheaper treatment options are frequently available.
- Make a referral to a home health-care agency in order to assist you and your family with wound management.

You and your team together can usually come up with a solution that you can afford and that helps to manage your wound.

Cultural Issues

Cultural or religious beliefs may prevent you from seeking appropriate medical attention or sticking with a wound treatment plan. Your wound team may not understand why you may not want to follow through with certain treatment recommendations—so discuss any concerns with your team. They can then take into account any of your cultural and religious beliefs in order to make sure that the treatment plan respects your beliefs. If you feel that your health-care team is not respecting your beliefs, find a different team.

Caregiving Issues

Caring for a wound, particularly one that is chronic or requires regular dressings or home treatments, may tax your energy or the energy of your caregiver, and may be very difficult for a person living alone. If you are not able to carry out your treatment plan, discuss this with your wound team. They may be able to simplify your regime, teach you easier techniques to apply a dressing, or arrange for home health-care visits. See Chapter 37 and Additional Resources for information on caregiving.

Life Goes On: Wounds That Can't Be Healed

There are some wounds, it may be eventually determined, that resist efforts to heal them. Wound healing may not be possible for everyone. Each wound is—as you are—unique.

Certain wounds may never heal. Sometimes the underlying cause of the wound can never be treated; for example, if you are very immobile and the pressure on your pressure ulcer can never be reduced, or if the blood flow to your wound is permanently extremely low. In these cases and others, the chances of healing are poor. Some people with chronic debilitating neurologic disorders, malnutrition, and immobility may have chronic wounds that never heal. Providing good local wound care, taking measures to manage any pain you may have, preventing infection, and preserving your comfort and quality of life then become the most important features of your wound management plan. Your wound team should speak to you and your family about these issues.

If the causes of your wound cannot be reduced or eliminated, your wound team will focus on your overall function, trying to get you back doing the things you like to do with the least amount of pain, odor, financial cost to you, and risk of infection. Everybody with a wound has unique requirements. We discuss these issues further in Chapter 31 ("Wounds in the Dying") and Chapter 34 ("Pain").

Before coming to the conclusion that your wound may not heal, your wound team will work with you to make sure that all the problems that can be treated have been treated properly.

When an Amputation Is Unavoidable

In people with diabetes, a foot ulcer, and high risk of infection, your doctor may suggest amputation. You may seek a second opinion, but if the consensus is still an amputation, you may actually have a better quality of life after this procedure. Studies show that some people with foot ulcers, who suffer greatly and are limited in their mobility, are more mobile and pain-free than they have been in a long time after an amputation and after a limb prosthesis has been fit. See Chapter 28 for more on skin and wound care following amputation.

PART SEVEN

Wound Treatments

Let the Healing Begin

Coping with the stress of having a wound is plenty to deal with. But figuring out how to properly care for it shouldn't be an additional burden. There are over one thousand dressings on the market so it can be very confusing to decide what to use.

Just because one dressing is newer or more expensive than another does not mean it is better—in fact, the opposite can often be true. Even though new products arrive almost daily, and others are updated or improved frequently, some of the older wound care options work best.

Keep in mind that dressings and other wound care products are tools that can promote healing, but they aren't the only tools you will need. What you put on the wound is often not nearly as important as managing the underlying cause of the wound (for example, poor blood circulation). A key element in all wound treatment plans is identifying and treating, when possible, the underlying causes. If the cause of the wound remains unaddressed, existing wounds won't heal and may worsen, or new wounds may develop. Unless other problems such as pressure relief, poor nutrition, and blood flow are also addressed, dressings alone won't heal the wound. We have discussed many of these problems in other chapters; for example, you can accomplish a lot by reducing pressure (by turning regularly or by using appropriate support surfaces) to help heal pressure ulcers. You can use proper footwear for diabetic foot ulcers. Leg swelling can be relieved by wearing compression bandaging or stockings. Once you have addressed the underlying reasons why the wound is not healing , the next step is deciding what to dress the wound with.

Your wound team will recommend strategies and products for cleaning your wound, and advise you on what dressings to use. In this section, we will explain the most common categories of wound dressings so you can better understand your treatment. The dressing that your wound team uses for you will most likely fit into one of these categories. See "Wound Cleansers and Dressings" in the back of the book for additional information.

18
What Do I Put on This Wound?

Treatment of all chronic wounds follows the same four basic steps—debridement*, moisture balance, wound protection, and nutrition. Your wound specialist may debride (remove) any dead tissue, provide a moist wound-healing environment through the use of proper dressings, protect the wound from further injury, and advise you on proper nutrition to aid wound healing.

Cleaning Your Wound

The first step to dressing your wound is proper cleansing. Wound cleaning is a very important step in the healing process because it gets rid of the dead tissue that harbors bacteria and slows wound healing. Flushing the wound or wiping it clean with sterile water or normal saline is the best method of cleaning most chronic wounds. Many commercial wound cleaners are somewhat toxic to cells in the wound bed; thus, their use can slow healing. If your wound team suggests that you clean the wound with sterile water, you can buy it or make it yourself. Normal saline is a sterile saltwater solution that you can buy in the drugstore without a prescription (usually in the eye care section with contact lens supplies). Or you can make saline solution yourself; simply boil tap water for ten minutes, add salt, and let it cool (covered) before you put it on the wound.

To clean the skin around the wound (but not the wound itself), use clean, warm water and mild soap (such as unscented Dove). Make sure you rinse off all of the soap.

How to Choose a Dressing

Deciding what dressing to put on the wound can be daunting.

Usually, your wound team will select a dressing that helps to keep your wound moist (without drenching it), because that is usually the best way to help you heal. An exception to this is arterial ulcers (see below).

Most often, your wound team will try to use dressings that can go two or more days without needing to be changed. This can help promote healing (since the frequent changing of dressings can remove fragile new skin as it tries to form), reduce the frequency of any pain associated with dressing changes, and, of course, reduce the hassle.

The dressing that is chosen depends on the condition of the ulcer. Your wound team will examine your wound and ask you questions to help them decide what dressings may be good options for you.

Is there a lot of drainage? If there is a great deal of drainage, your wound team will select a dressing that is absorbent, so you don't have to change the dressing as often. Examples of dressings that are absorbent include foams (absorbent sponge-like dressings) and alginates. Alginate dressings are made from seaweed and are very absorptive. As drainage from the wound is absorbed, the surrounding skin is protected from getting too wet (too much wetness would slow healing, irritate the skin, and may cause your wound to get larger).

Q: TRUE OR FALSE: Leaving your chronic wound open to air (without a dressing) improves healing.
A: FALSE!
A chronic wound can develop an infection if left open to the microorganisms that are present in the air. Your wound is also susceptible to trauma if not protected. In addition, properly selected wound dressings can help heal the tissue in a wound. Air can't do this.

Green Drainage

Sometimes when there is a lot of green drainage coming from your wound, it can mean that your wound is infected by a certain type of bacteria called *Pseudomonas*. This can be treated with (1) dressings applied to the wound, (2) antibiotics given in pill form or intravenously, or (3) cleansing the wound with a solution of nine parts sterile water and one part white kitchen vinegar.

Is there a potential for infection? In reality, any open wound has the possibility of getting infected. As a result, many wound dressings have antibacterial properties. These dressings help prevent or help manage infection and control any odor. One example of an ingredient that is popular in many wound dressings is silver, which kills bacteria. Unlike antibiotics that you take by mouth, you are unlikely to develop a resistance to silver and very few people are allergic to it. Iodine is another ingredient in some wound dressings that is antibacterial.

Is there some dead tissue in the wound? If the wound contains any dead tissue (often yellow or black), it usually needs to be removed. Your wound team may do this using scissors or a scalpel if it is not too painful for you. Another method is to use dressings capable of removing the dead tissue. Many gel dressings are able to clean out (or debride) this dead tissue.

Is the wound deep? If the wound is more than just a surface wound, it usually needs to be "packed," meaning that the dressing needs to be pushed all the way to the bottom of the wound and come out on top. This loosely fills the wound so it does not close on the surface, leaving an open hole underneath that could potentially fill with infection. Packing the wound enables it to heal from the bottom up, and from the inside out. It is important to "fluff, not stuff" the packing—the wound should be packed loosely so that the healing tissue does not have too much pressure on it. Having too much pressure in the wound may make the wound bigger. Not all dressings are appropriate for packing.

Do you have pain in or near the wound? Some wounds are very painful, particularly when the dressing is changed. There are many newer dressings that can be much less painful than others. One type of dressing, for example, uses soft silicone rather than harsher adhesive materials; therefore, it is very gentle on the skin and does not tear when coming off. Some dressings also have painkillers in the dressing.

What if your wound has one or more of the above characteristics? It is very common for a wound to have one or more qualities that can complicate management (for example, an infection and a lot of drainage). In this case, you need a dressing that can perform one or more functions. Many such hybrid or all-in-one dressings exist. One example of such a dressing is silver foam, which helps absorb drainage and kills bacteria.

Who will be doing the dressing changes: you, a family member, or a home health nurse? This is an important point to consider because certain dressings are more difficult to apply than others. Sometimes family members are ashamed to admit that they are uncomfortable dressing

 Why Not Use Plain Gauze Rather than a Fancy Dressing?

Plain gauze does not have any antibacterial properties, so if your wound has an infection, gauze will not help. Gauze can also stick to the wound, making it painful to remove. Gauze can also leave some cotton residue in the wound, again making it more likely to get infected. However, gauze can still be used to cover another dressing. Many dressings on the market are much better options than gauze alone, and they are often affordable.

the wound. It is important that the wound team know about this, however, so that the wound can be dressed appropriately. Never dress a wound unless you are completely comfortable in doing so. When you speak with your wound team, don't be afraid to tell them if you or a family member is not comfortable applying a certain type of dressing. A dressing that is easier to use can often be found, or the team can help you better understand how to apply it.

Is the wound in the leg or foot, and do you know how good your blood flow is? If you have very poor blood flow in the area of the wound, keeping the wound moist may make it worse, more painful, and more susceptible to infection. For this type of wound, it is most important to use a dressing that is antimicrobial but keeps the wound dry. An example of this type of dressing is povidone-iodine, an antiseptic.

19
Growth Factors and Engineered Skin
The Future Is Here

Over the past few years, technologically advanced dressings (called biological dressings*) have become available. Some of these dressings sound like they came right out of science fiction: some look and function like skin but are made from pig membranes; some skin substitutes are made from actual living skin cells, skin growth-enhancing factors, and so on. These dressings can function like skin grafts, except that you don't have to go through surgery.

Biological dressings require a noninfected wound with healthy tissue. However, they can get infected so you may need an antimicrobial dressing in addition to the biological dressing. Biological dressings can cause allergic reactions and are very expensive. Also, because biological dressings are from an animal or human, eventually the body will reject a biological dressing. If this happens and your wound is not yet healed, then you may need to use a nonbiological dressing or require a surgical skin graft. Also, the use of pig, other animal, or human components may not align with some religious beliefs.

Biological dressings can sometimes shorten healing times. Research is ongoing in the area of biological dressings and more research is needed to see which biologic dressings are worth the high cost, and which specific types of wound these dressings work best on. The biological dressings most commonly used in wound treatment include growth factors and living skin equivalents. In this chapter, we will explain what these therapies are and how they work. See Appendix for more information.

Growth Factors

Growth factors play an important role in the healing process by stimulating tissue cells to grow and multiply (Table 5). If the body doesn't produce and remove various growth factors with correct timing, the wound healing process can get stuck. This leaves the wound caught between stages of healing instead of following the normal healing process.

In the past decade, growth factors have been studied to determine exactly how they function in healing and how they may be used in the treatment of chronic wounds. The only synthetic growth factor currently approved by the U.S. Food and Drug Administration (FDA) for use in wound care is platelet-derived growth factor (PDGF, brand name Regranex), which is thought to induce fibroblasts (components of healthy wound healing tissue) to multiply and collagen to form. PDGF is recommended for use on diabetic foot ulcers that have

Table 5: What Do the Growth Factors Do?

Type	Description
TGF-B (transforming growth factor beta)	Controls movement of cells to sites of inflammation
bFGF (basic fibroblast growth factor)	Stimulates the growth of blood vessels (also called angiogenesis)
VEGF (vascular endothelial growth factor)	Stimulates the growth of blood vessels (also called angiogenesis)
IGF (insulin-like growth factor)	Increases collagen synthesis
EGF (epidermal growth factor)	Stimulates skin regeneration

adequate blood flow. It should not be used on infected wounds or in people with poor blood supply to their legs. A dime-size thickness of PDGF can be applied to wounds using a sterile applicator, such as a swab, and the wound can then be dressed with a saline-moistened gauze.

Other growth factors have been tested or are undergoing testing in clinical trials but are not yet approved for use in wound care (TGF-B, bFGF, and EGF among them).

Living Skin Equivalents

Living skin equivalents are also called tissue-engineered skin substitutes. These products are expensive and require special storage, and some expire quickly. They are derived from biological substances, such as bovine (cow) collagen and human newborn foreskin. All skin substitutes should be used on wounds with good blood flow that are free from infection, and avoided in people with allergies to bovine products. Several applications may be needed. This sterile procedure, which can usually be done in an outpatient clinic setting, requires special training.

Table 6: Living Skin Substitutes

	What it replaces	What it's made from	What it's used for
Dermagraft	Dermis (bottom layer of the skin)	• Human fibroblasts on a polyglactin mesh	• Burns • Diabetic foot ulcers
Apligraf	Epidermis and dermis (top and bottom layer of the skin)	• Type 1 collagen • Human fibroblasts • Human keratinocytes	• Venous ulcers • Diabetic foot ulcers

Two living skin substitutes approved by the FDA in the United States are Dermagraft and Apligraf.

Dermagraft is a single layer of human newborn cells on a mesh of dissolvable suture material. The cells secrete and fill in the mesh with a substance that helps healing. Dermagraft is used to treat patients with burns and diabetic foot ulcers.

Apligraf is a two-layer skin substitute containing human newborn cells as well as collagen and human keratinocytes (the cells that synthesize keratin, which is a key component of skin). Apligraf is FDA-approved for use in both venous and diabetic foot ulcers. When applied to venous ulcers, Apligraf should be used in addition to compression therapy. If you have a diabetic foot ulcer, appropriate off-loading devices are also used.

Your wound care team will help advise you on whether living skin substitutes are appropriate in your case, and if so, which substitute would be right for you. Table 6 provides brief descriptions of what they are. Your wound team can help you decide.

20

Adjunctive and Alternative Therapies

A wide variety of wound care aids and products you put on the skin are available to enhance dressings and are used in addition to traditional therapies.

There is not a lot of strong medical evidence that supports using these sometimes expensive products to heal wounds, but you and your wound team may decide in some cases that they are right for you. Sometimes it may be worth trying a product or device for a couple of weeks to see if there is an improvement in your wound. Remember that addressing the cause of the wound is far more likely to help heal your wound than adjunctive therapies. In this chapter we explain a few such therapies in case your wound team and you are considering one or more of them.

Vacuum Therapy

Vacuum therapy (Figure 22) uses negative air pressure to promote wound closure. This system consists of a foam dressing cut to the size of the wound, a vacuum tube, and a vacuum pump. One end of the vacuum tube is placed over the foam dressing and the other end connects to the vacuum pump. The dressing is sealed securely in place with adhesive tape. The pump removes drainage from the wound. This process may reduce bacteria and promote healing. Special training is required to operate this device. Vacuum devices can be used while you are in the hospital, or at home by home care agencies.

Vacuum therapy is most useful in wounds that drain large amounts of fluids; in wounds after they have been surgically debrided; or in

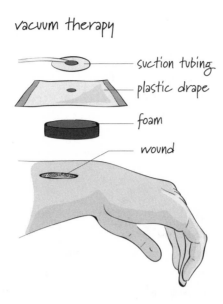

vacuum therapy

suction tubing
plastic drape
foam
wound

Figure 22: Vacuum therapy uses negative air pressure to promote wound closure.

postoperative wounds. Vacuum therapy should not be used when there is bone infection (osteomyelitis), cancer, or dead tissue or fistulas in the wound.

The vacuum tube can be quite long (up to five or six feet), which means you need to either stay in one place or carry the unit with you. Depending on your response to the therapy, your health-care team may suggest that you use vacuum therapy for several weeks. A smaller, portable version of vacuum therapy is available and runs on rechargeable batteries with a smaller drainage capacity. Keep in mind that incorrect use of the vacuum device, such as lying on the tubing or improperly setting the pressure, can result in a new or worsening wound.

Warming Therapy

Warming therapy, also called noncontact normothermic wound therapy, involves a dressing which increases the temperature of the wound and may improve blood flow to the wound. This therapy may help to heal chronic wounds that have not healed using more traditional therapies, and have low blood flow, such as arterial ulcers or some diabetic foot ulcers. Warming therapy should not be used on third-degree burns. Also, it requires skill to apply and you need to understand how to manage the heat properly so the wound or surrounding skin is not damaged further.

Hydrotherapy

Hydrotherapy, one of the oldest therapies for wound healing, can take various forms, including pulsatile lavage (which cleans the wound by irrigating it with normal saline under pressure), whirlpool therapy, or irrigation with a syringe. As with most treatments, the type of therapy used depends on your wound type. Whirlpool therapy may result in a very wet, possibly infected wound and should not be used in wounds with poor blood flow (arterial wounds).

Therapeutic Light

Sometimes light or its energy is used to help heal a wound. Therapeutic light treatments include ultraviolet (UV) energy and laser therapy.

Although not a form of light, UV energy is usually categorized as a therapeutic light therapy. UV energy lies between X-rays and visible light on the electromagnetic spectrum. UV radiation may enhance wound cleaning and may help infected wounds. It should not be used in people with certain chronic conditions such as diabetes or heart, kidney, or liver disease.

Lasers may regenerate nerves and help wounds heal. They may also be helpful in reducing pain.

Ultrasound

Ultrasound waves are sound waves that may help wounds heal by improving collagen secretion. Collagen is essential to wound healing and improving blood flow. Ultrasound should not be used over areas with no blood flow or over dead tissue.

Electrical Stimulation

Electrical stimulation is delivered through electrodes that are applied to the skin. It is thought to improve blood flow and destroy microorganisms, as well as reduce pain. It should not be used over an area with cancer or over infected bone (osteomyelitis).

Hyperbaric Oxygen Therapy

Hyperbaric oxygen therapy (HBOT) delivers 100 percent oxygen to your wound. Increasing the amount of oxygen in the blood may help white blood cells fight infection and may improve blood flow to the wound. HBOT also increases levels of nitric oxide, which increases blood flow. Improved blood flow may result in better delivery of nutrients to the wound and improved wound healing. Usually, for HBOT your entire body is placed in an enclosed chamber. Possible uses for HBOT include venous stasis ulcers and diabetic foot ulcers.

Newer Therapies

Several new therapies for wound care have been developed in the past decade. These newer therapies may help to stimulate cells required for wound healing. Treatment with monochromatic near-infrared photo energy (MIRE) is approved by the FDA for increasing circulation and reducing pain. Cell proliferation induction (CPI) technology uses a radiofrequency signal to stimulate wound healing. It may increase cell growth, especially in pressure ulcers. In mist ultrasound transport therapy (MIST), a sterile saline mist transfers ultrasound energy to the wound. MIST may decrease bacteria, reduce the amount of dead tissue, increase collagen, and improve blood flow.

21

Surgery for Chronic
Wound Treatment
When Cutting Can Heal

Most wounds will heal without requiring surgery. Minor procedures, such as cleaning out your wound, are not usually considered surgery, and can typically be done by your wound care team at the bedside or in the office. Sometimes, however, the best way to facilitate healing is through major surgery. Wounds such as pressure ulcers, venous ulcers, and arterial ulcers may benefit from surgery.

You and your wound need to be a good fit for surgery in order for you to derive benefits from the operation (see box). For example, surgery that is done to heal a pressure ulcer can fail over 50 percent of the time. Therefore, the surgeon must be very careful when deciding which patients will benefit from surgery, to increase the odds of healing. A surgeon will take into account many factors to decide whether you are a good candidate.

If you are a good candidate for surgery, you may do very well with the procedure and have a high likelihood of healing completely. When a wound undergoes surgery, a new acute wound is created when all the infected, dead, or scarred tissue is removed. During surgery, skin and tissues (which include the blood vessels, tendons, and muscles) are transferred from a particular location to the area of the wound: the skin

Could Surgery Be the Answer for You?

Whether or not surgery will help you to heal depends on a number of factors:

1. *Your overall health.* Surgery can sometimes result in quite a lot of blood loss as well as postoperative immobility, so the surgeon needs to make sure he or she is operating on someone who can get through these stresses. The surgeon will also consider what other medical conditions you have.

2. *Your ulcer's depth.* Usually only very deep ulcers (into the muscle or deeper) are considered for surgery. Bone infection will also be a consideration when a surgeon is deciding if surgery is appropriate.

3. *Your wound's cause.* If this is a diabetic foot ulcer or a pressure ulcer, are you able to reduce pressure from the wound at all? Can any infection in the wound be treated? Postsurgical wounds may also be treated with further surgery.

4. *How you follow medical advice.* If you have stuck to your wound team's recommendations in the past (for example, tried to stay off the wound and used the recommended treatment), you're a better candidate.

continued

continues

5. *How many ulcers you have.* If you have more than
   one pressure ulcer, you may not be a candidate
   for surgery. Or if you have many diabetic foot
   ulcers, you might be a better candidate for an
   amputation.

6. *Your surgical history.* How many surgeries have
   you had in the past to treat an ulcer in the same
   location? Usually if you have had more than
   one previous surgery, you may not heal well if
   you have another surgery due to the scar tissue
   (which is never as strong as unscarred tissue) that
   remains in the area.

and tissues that are transferred are called a "flap" or "graft." Six weeks
after successful surgery, 60 percent of the strength of the wound site is
usually regained.

The type of surgeon who repairs wounds is usually a plastic
surgeon, a surgeon who repairs blood flow to a wound is a vascular
surgeon, and a surgeon who repairs foot deformities is an orthopedic
surgeon or podiatrist.

Surgery for Pressure Ulcers

There are many types of surgical flaps that a plastic surgeon may
choose to perform to help heal a pressure ulcer.

Surgery for Foot and Leg Ulcers Caused by Poor Blood Flow

We discussed ulcers primarily caused by poor blood flow in Chapter 11. Poor blood flow may be a secondary cause in other types of ulcers, such as pressure ulcers, diabetic foot ulcers, and venous stasis ulcers.

Surgery for blood flow impairment in the lower legs has become much more common over the past few years with many new, less invasive procedures. After your wound team has determined that you have blood flow impairment to your legs (you may have had one of the tests described in Chapter 11), you may be referred to a vascular surgeon. Your vascular surgeon may then decide, after discussion with you, to do an arteriogram. An arteriogram is a test where dye is injected—usually into a blood vessel in your groin—and X-rays are taken to see if the dye goes to all your major blood vessels and if there are any blockages. If blockages in a blood vessel are found, your surgeon may decide that one of the following procedures may be right for you:

- *Angioplasty.* This is also known as a "balloon" procedure. The vascular surgeon will first inject some freezing solution into the skin in your groin area. Then, he or she will insert a catheter into a blood vessel in your groin, push it farther down into the blood vessel, and inflate a balloon in the area of the blockage. This opens up the blockage, and sometimes a stent (something that holds the blood vessel open even after the balloon is removed) is placed. This is usually an outpatient procedure, meaning you do not need to be admitted to the hospital or stay overnight. The up side to angioplasty is that even if you have medical problems that may prevent you from having surgery, you may still be able to have an angioplasty. The down side is that a vessel that is opened up with a balloon may not stay open as long as with arterial bypass surgery.

- *Arterial bypass surgery*. Arterial bypass surgery may be the best way to restore arterial flow in some people. The type and extent of bypass surgery depends on the ulcer's severity and location, as well as your general health. It is major surgery done in the operating room under a general anesthetic and so has risks associated with it, as with any surgery. You need to be medically healthy (usually meaning no major heart or lung problems that would prevent you from going under a general anesthetic) to have this surgery.

Surgery for Venous Leg Ulcers

Venous ulcers can be managed without surgery most of the time. There are two types of surgery that may help heal venous stasis ulcers.

- *Vein stripping*. This can help certain people with recurrent venous stasis ulcers. Usually, people that are relatively young (in their forties or younger), with ulcers that have recurred for years despite treatment with compression, may do well with this surgery. A vascular surgeon usually performs vein surgery.

- *Skin grafts or flaps*. Skin grafting can be successful for some people with venous ulcers, or injuries caused by burns, trauma, or surgery. It is performed by a surgeon, usually a plastic surgeon. The surgeon may choose skin grafting as the preferred treatment option if the wound is not healing on its own and there is good blood flow to the wound. Skin grafting is a process in which your surgeon takes (or "harvests") a paper-thin layer of skin and attaches it to your wound site. Your surgeon will make sure that the "donor" site (usually the thigh) has enough blood flow so it can heal on its own. Depending on what type of graft you need, it may be applied under either local (where the area is frozen with a needle but you are not put to sleep) or general anesthesia (where you are

How Are Your Veins?

Your surgeon needs to make sure that you have problems with the superficial veins only, because if you have a problem with the deep veins, and the superficial veins are stripped, it may make your ulcers worse.

put to sleep). Sometimes, the skin graft can be performed as an outpatient procedure with no need to stay in the hospital overnight.

It takes up to three weeks to develop 30 percent of the normal skin strength at the wound site, and up to six months for 90 percent of the strength to be regained. Sometimes, it may appear that the skin graft has taken, but then failed—however, this may be because the graft did not "take" fully to begin with. So once you start moving your limb again after the surgery, remember that it may take several weeks or even months for complete healing to take place.

The success or failure of any skin graft depends on how much blood flow is in and around the wound. The graft will die if there is insufficient blood flow. The skin graft can take anywhere from three days to two weeks to develop new blood vessels and start to settle in.

Surgery for Foot Ulcers in Diabetes

The most significant risks that lead to foot wounds in people with diabetes are neuropathy and foot deformity. Foot deformity results from the neuropathy and joint abnormality, which can result in "clawed toes" and increased pressure beneath the base of the toes. Many people with

diabetes and foot ulcers also have blood flow problems and may also
need surgery to improve their blood flow (see above). Two types of doctors operate on the feet of people with diabetes: orthopedic surgeons
(medical doctors who also do several years of residency to train as orthopedic specialists, and may train specifically as foot and ankle specialists) and podiatrists (who train in a doctorate program in podiatric
medicine and have further training involving foot and ankle surgery).
Whoever you see, make sure it is someone you trust and feel comfortable with (just like when you seek any health-care professional).

Years ago, orthopedic surgeons and podiatrists managed diabetic
foot ulcers by local debridement, antibiotics, and amputation. These
days, amputations should not be necessary except for severe foot ulcers that are at high risk for blood infection. In the past twenty years,
orthopedic surgeons have been able to help change the problem areas
of a foot (also known as foot "reconstruction") in a person with diabetes, and thus help prevent ulcers from forming, and also heal any
existing ulcers. Some types of surgeries that an orthopedic surgeon or
podiatrist may do include:

- *Local debridement.* If there is an infection in the bone that
  cannot be treated with antibiotics, the surgeon may be able to
  use local freezing and clean out the bone by scraping away the
  infected parts.

- *Release of contractures.* This procedure can help correct foot
  deformities such as clawed toes, shown in Figure 23.

- *Exostectomies.* This procedure involves removal of bony prominences that stick out, cause pressure, and don't allow wounds
  to heal.

- *Arthrodesis.* This procedure involves joint fusion to correct
  deformity.

All of these surgical reconstructive procedures are aimed at decreasing pressure over the area at risk. Surgery may also make the foot

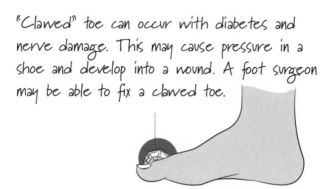

"Clawed" toe can occur with diabetes and nerve damage. This may cause pressure in a shoe and develop into a wound. A foot surgeon may be able to fix a clawed toe.

Figure 23: Clawed toes.

a more normal shape so that it can be managed and kept ulcer-free with custom-made shoes and/or braces. Some of these orthopedic procedures can be done by freezing the nerves in the feet so you don't need to be put under a general anesthetic for the procedure.

Complications that can potentially occur after foot surgery include infection, hardware failure, recurrent ulcers, and amputation. However, the prevention of amputation is achieved about 90 percent of the time.

After the Operation

Most postoperative wounds will usually heal if there is enough blood flow. Good postoperative care is crucial to ensure that you heal well, without complications. These days, with shorter hospital stays, you and your loved one may need to do quite a lot of postoperative care yourselves to help ensure that your wound heals properly.

Potential complications after surgery include excessive bleeding, wound separation, and infection. To try to prevent these complications from occurring, it is crucial to follow your surgeon's team's suggestions on how to position yourself. For example, after a skin graft is placed, you usually need to immobilize the wound site for a while to allow it

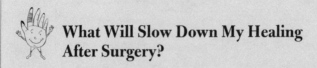 **What Will Slow Down My Healing After Surgery?**

- *Smoking.* Smoking decreases blood flow and oxygen. Stopping smoking four to six weeks before surgery can make a big difference in how well you will do. Continuing to *not* smoke after surgery also promotes wound healing.

- *Spasticity.* Permanently contracted joints can slow wound healing if they impair your ability to reposition yourself.

- *Poor nutrition.* Eating properly is very important. If you are not able to eat well, nutritional supplements (by mouth, or through intravenous or gastric tubes) may be necessary.

- *Incontinence.* Both bowel and bladder incontinence can contaminate the surgical site if it is near the buttocks.

- *Infection.* Any infection in the deep tissues or bones should be treated before the operation if possible.

- *Diabetes.* Persons with diabetes are more likely to have poor wound healing due in part to a delayed immune response and increased risk of infection. Poor wound healing is even more likely to occur in people with diabetes if blood sugar is not well controlled and particularly if it is consistently too high. Therefore, after the operation, it is very important that close monitoring of your blood glucose takes place and good control is maintained.

continued

continues

- *Alcohol intake.* Excessive alcohol intake can impair the immune system, lead to malnutrition, and cause liver damage.

- *Medications.* Many over-the-counter medications (such as aspirin and related drugs) and herbal supplements may slow wound healing. Tell your surgeon exactly what you are taking, especially if it is not a prescription medication.

to heal. Moving it too much may disrupt the skin graft and cause it to slide or separate from the wound site.

You may be seen by a physiotherapist and occupational therapist after the operation, and they can give you direction with respect to this. Additionally, it is very important that your nutrition is good. You may also be seen by a dietician in the hospital who can guide you on what to eat and any supplements you should be taking to help the healing process.

PART EIGHT

Wounds in Specific Populations and Conditions

22

Nervous System Damage
*Spinal Cord Injury, Spina Bifida,
and Multiple Sclerosis*

*Mr. J is a thirty-nine-year-old man who has been paralyzed since he
was nineteen and had a fall when working on a fishing boat. Nonethe-
less he is an active man who really enjoys life. Three months ago, he
developed a pressure ulcer on his buttocks, which has turned his life
upside down. He has stopped working in order to make healing this
ulcer his top priority. As a result he is not spending as much time with
his friends as he was before and is starting to feel depressed. We knew
that things had to change for Mr. J quickly.*

When it is functioning normally, the skin's jobs include sweating
(to help with cooling and regulating your body's temperature) and
normal sensation (for example, feeling pain, burning, and pressure).
Nerves transmit messages from the brain and spinal cord (together
called the central nervous system) to the skin and carry messages from
the skin back to the spinal cord and brain.

When these nerves are damaged (such as in spinal cord injury,
spina bifida, or multiple sclerosis), the skin cannot do its jobs as well as
it should. As a result, if you have nervous system damage, you need to
take extra care of your skin, otherwise serious problems could result.

In this chapter, we will explain in more detail why you are at risk for skin problems, and help you find ways to keep you and your skin feeling good.

Why Am I at Risk for Skin Problems?

Decreased Awareness of Sensations

As illustrated in Figure 24, when you have had an injury to your spinal cord, you may have reduced or no skin sensation below the level of injury. You may not be able to feel or move below this level of injury, so you are more likely to sit or lie for long periods of time on certain parts

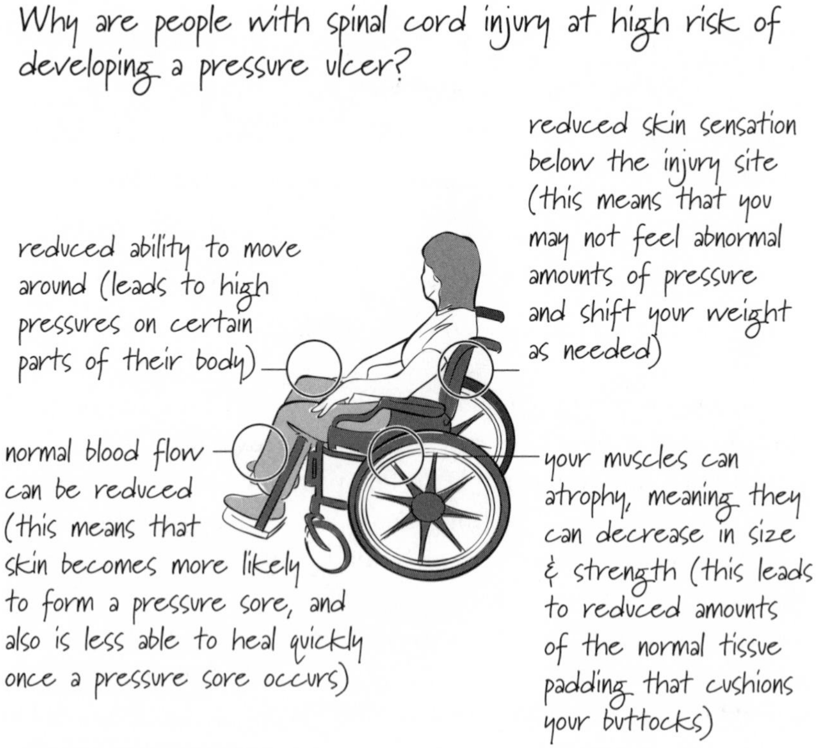

Why are people with spinal cord injury at high risk of developing a pressure ulcer?

reduced skin sensation below the injury site (this means that you may not feel abnormal amounts of pressure and shift your weight as needed)

reduced ability to move around (leads to high pressures on certain parts of their body)

normal blood flow can be reduced (this means that skin becomes more likely to form a pressure sore, and also is less able to heal quickly once a pressure sore occurs)

your muscles can atrophy, meaning they can decrease in size & strength (this leads to reduced amounts of the normal tissue padding that cushions your buttocks)

Figure 24: Spinal cord injury and pressure ulcer risk.

of your body. The longer you stay in one position without moving, the more the blood flow in your skin is reduced because of the prolonged pressure on the area. In addition, the amount of muscle (which helps cushion your buttocks) may be reduced because of the spinal cord injury. The combination of reduced sensation, reduced muscle cushioning, and long periods of pressure can lead to skin breakdown and development of pressure sores. Pressure sores may even be life threatening but are frequently preventable.

Decreased Blood Flow

People who have had an injury to their nervous system are more likely to get edema, which is swelling caused by pooling of your body fluids in the tissues under the skin, especially in your legs when you have been sitting up for a long time. Because your mobility may be more limited than if you did not have nervous system damage, your blood doesn't circulate as well. When pressure sores do happen, your skin is slower to heal because spinal cord injury often results in less blood flow to the skin.

One way you can reduce your swelling is to stretch your muscles and exercise. Raising your arms from time to time above your head can help keep fluid from pooling. Talk to a physiotherapist about the right level of activity and best exercises for you.

Edema in your legs that gets worse when you have been sitting can often be prevented by using compression stockings (see Chapter 12).

Don't smoke! The nicotine in cigarettes results in your blood vessels getting narrower, and so prevents adequate blood and oxygen from flowing normally.

Spasms

Spasms can occur with nervous system damage because the nerves can misfire signals to the muscles, causing them to contract even when you did not want them to. These spasms can result in your skin rubbing against your wheelchair or bed, causing shear and friction, and can increase your risk of skin breakdown.

Sweating

Any injury to your spinal cord can also stop you from sweating below the site of the injury. You may also have increased sweating above the injury site, often in your chest and face. As a result, you need to be careful in keeping your body temperature within the normal range. Abnormal sweating also puts you at risk for developing skin irritation and fungal infections, which we talk about later in this chapter.

Types of Skin Problems in Nervous System Injuries

Table 7 lists the kinds of wounds most commonly seen among those with nervous system injuries.

Pressure Ulcers

A pressure ulcer is caused by continuous pressure that damages the skin and tissues underneath. The first sign of a pressure ulcer forming is a

Table 7: Nervous System Injuries: What Am I at Risk For?

Wound Issue	Spinal cord injury	Spina bifida	Multiple sclerosis
Pressure ulcers	√	√	√
Skin irritation due to incontinence	√	√	√
Fungal skin infections	√	√	
Sources of pressure frequently include ill-fitting braces and bony deformities		√	
Ulcers at medication injection sites			√

red area of skin that does not go away. The good news is that there is a lot you can do for yourself or your loved one to prevent pressure ulcers and help them heal faster if they occur. If you see a red area of skin, relieve the pressure by getting your weight off the area. You should stay off the area until it clears. If the red area does not clear within twenty-four hours, call your health-care professional. If you have any open areas on your skin, stay off the area and call a health-care professional immediately.

You can greatly reduce your risk of developing a pressure sore by shifting sitting positions. Use special pressure-reducing booties to protect vulnerable areas such as your heels. You could also keep your heels off the bed (use a pillow or two under your lower legs). If a pressure sore develops, remove all pressure immediately to keep the sore from worsening and getting deeper. See Part II for more about the prevention and treatment of pressure sores.

Burns and Rashes

You may also be at risk of burns because of your skin's reduced ability to feel sensations. Treatment for burns is the same for people with nerve injuries as for anyone (see Chapter 14).

Increased moisture due to sweating can cause skin rashes. Rashes can also be caused by urinary incontinence, tapes, soaps, fabrics, or anything else that irritates the skin. Increased moisture can also result in rashes due to fungal skin infections. Rashes due to skin irritants or fungus are often very easy to treat with a prescription cream (see Chapter 35). If you have a rash from head to toe, it may be due to an allergy to a medication. Keep the skin clean and dry and contact your health-care provider.

Keeping Your Skin Healthy

Inspect Your Skin

The best way for you to tell if your skin is healthy is to inspect it at least once a day (and preferably twice), particularly in areas where you have decreased sensation, where bones protrude below the skin (see

Chapter 5, Figure 5 for common areas that pressure ulcers can develop in), and where you have had pressure sores in the past.

It's easiest to perform your skin inspection when you are undressed anyway; for example, before or after you bathe. Look for any red marks, rashes, blisters, scrapes, bruises, or indentations from elastic (indentations are a clue that there is too much pressure on the area). Use a mirror or ask a loved one to inspect if you can't see some parts of your body. Specially designed mirrors are available to help you do this. Also check your toes for any redness around the nails or ingrown toenails. One way to prevent ingrown nails is to cut your nails straight across. If you notice any redness or ingrown nails, call your health-care provider.

There's a Right Way to Wash

Here are some tips on cleaning your skin properly to reduce your risk of skin breakdown:

- Minimize use of soaps labeled "antibacterial" or "antimicrobial." They can prevent the skin from fighting infection the way it should.
- Avoid products that make the skin too dry (for example, harsh soaps or lotions containing alcohol).
- Use a gentle, fragrance-free moisturizer (such as Eucerin) after you bathe.
- Avoid using talc powders. Sometime fungal infections can develop in areas where talc is used. Talc powders can also become "cakey" and keep too much moisture on the skin, resulting in skin breakdown.

Skin folds, such as in the groin area and underarms, may develop rashes easily because of the increased moisture and warmth. You may need to wash them more than once a day to keep them clean and dry. Increasing the air circulation to these areas to help prevent rashes can be accomplished by positioning the arms and legs so the skin surfaces are separated.

Clean up any urine and stool incontinence quickly—otherwise, they can irritate the skin and cause skin breakdown.

Always check the fit of your clothes, shoes, and equipment to be certain that they are not too tight.

Change Positions

Change your body positioning frequently so you relieve pressure over bony areas. Change positions every fifteen minutes, shift your weight from one side of the buttocks to the other, and turn frequently in bed (at least every two hours if you can manage it).

In a wheelchair, push straight up, lean side to side, bending forward over your knees, recline the seat of your electric wheelchair, or have someone tilt you back in your manual chair. Always use a proper wheelchair cushion.

In bed, pad bony areas at risk for pressure sore formation (such as your hips) with pillows. Keep a pillow between your knees while you are on your side.

Reduce Your Risk of Burns

Because your sensation may be decreased, it is important to be alert for potential exposure to burns.

- Wear sunscreen when out in the sun.
- Avoid hot items (such as hot water bottles and electric blankets) on areas where you have no sensation.
- Check the temperature of bath and shower water carefully before bathing.

Reduce Stress

Stress, worry, anxiety, and depression can result in your losing interest and paying less attention to your skin care (for more information on these issues, see Chapter 2). Speak to your health-care team candidly about your feelings so they can help you find ways to improve your care for your skin—and your outlook.

Are You Using the Right Equipment?

Here are some questions to ask to ensure that the equipment you are using fits properly and reduces your chances of developing pressure sores:

- *Wheelchair*: Does your wheelchair support your back? Are your footrests placed in the correct position, and at the right height? Are you using the best wheelchair cushion? Have your wheelchair cushion assessed at least once every two years.
- *Bed*: Are you using a good mattress? Your health-care team can arrange for an occupational therapist to come to your home and look at your bed and other equipment you may have.
- *Urinary catheters*: Is the correct size being used? Is it being changed frequently enough? Are the straps of any leg bags used too tight? Make sure you check your skin underneath the catheters.
- *Arm/leg splints and braces*: Do any splints or braces you may be using fit properly? Make sure to check your skin after using them.

Spina Bifida

The term *spina bifida* comes from Latin and literally means "split" or "open" spine. Spina bifida is a condition that develops at the end of the first month of pregnancy, and results because the two sides of the embryo's spine do not join together, leaving an open area. No one knows exactly why spina bifida occurs, although we do know that it is associated with low folic acid levels in the mother during the first trimester of pregnancy.

Of the several types of spina bifida, the form that involves serious nervous system damage is spina bifida myelomeningocele, in which the spinal cord pushes through a hole in the back. There is damage to the spinal cord, so an individual born with this type of spina bifida usually has some paralysis, and problems with bladder and bowel control. The higher the opening is on the back, the more severe the paralysis is.

People with spina bifida and paralysis are at the same risks for skin problems as those with any other type of paralysis, including pressure ulcers, skin irritation from incontinence, and fungal infection. They should maintain rigorous skin care, as explained above in the spinal cord injury section.

There are some unique situations in spina bifida that can lead to pressure sores. People with spina bifida may be more likely to use leg braces, so make sure that the braces have been fitted for you properly. Also, bone deformities, particularly in the spine and feet, can lead to pressure sores. Make sure you have been fitted for proper shoes, and protect your feet while swimming (check with your foot specialist about water exercise shoes). Wear footwear at all times when not in a bed or chair. Also, it may be tempting, with paralysis in spina bifida, to crawl from place to place for a short distance. This is not a good idea, as pressure sores can easily develop.

Multiple Sclerosis

Multiple sclerosis (MS) is an autoimmune disorder in which the immune system (the system in your body that fights infection) attacks the body's nerves. A person with MS can have many symptoms: decreased sensation, paralysis, and impaired bowel and bladder function. Not everyone with MS has all these symptoms, but having them increases your risk of developing skin breakdown, just like those who have other causes of paralysis.

People with MS also are at risk of developing ulcers at the sites where they give themselves medication injections. After months or years of injections in the same site, the skin and tissues of the area can scar and break down. Once this happens, the wound can be very slow to heal because of the scar tissue in the area. For this reason it is important to rotate injection sites.

Mr. J was looking depressed when he came to our clinic. As we discussed his situation with him, we realized that he was not taking advantage of all the resources available. We were able to identify sources of funding which allowed him to buy optimal bed and wheelchair surfaces. Mr. J was also eligible to have someone come into his home to do some of the housecleaning. With this extra help, Mr. J was able to maintain a better balance between exercise and rest. He also decided that it was time to stop smoking and start eating better. Mr. J wanted to heal this wound so he could go back to work and go back to his old life.

It did take time, but six months later, Mr. J went back to work. He also returned to his active social schedule and has regained his bright outlook on life.

23
Healing Challenges and the Older Person

Chronic wounds are more common in older people than in those who are younger. People over the age of eighty-five are the fastest-growing segment of the older adult population. About half of people over the age of eighty-five live in long-term care facilities (nursing homes), and the other half live at home.

The reason that chronic wounds are more common in the elderly is that normal wound healing tends to slow with age and with chronic diseases such as diabetes, dementia, and stroke. However, with good care, these older adults with wounds do just as well as younger people do.

Aging, Skin, and Wound Healing

As people get older, several changes occur that make wounds slower to heal than they once did (Figure 25). For example, if you bump your leg against a shopping cart or a wheelchair, the fragile outer layer of skin may tear, and the resultant wound may be slow to heal. With increased age, your skin can become thinner and drier, so it requires more care and moisture (see the section on "Dry Skin" in Chapter 35). An older person with a wound may be more prone to developing an infection because our immune systems change as we get older, which can slow the healing of a wound.

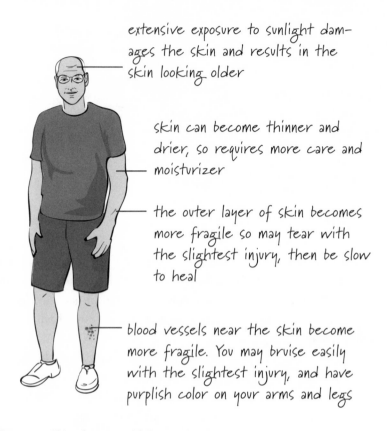

extensive exposure to sunlight damages the skin and results in the
skin looking older

skin can become thinner and
drier, so requires more care and
moisturizer

the outer layer of skin becomes
more fragile so may tear with
the slightest injury, then be slow
to heal

blood vessels near the skin become
more fragile. You may bruise easily
with the slightest injury, and have
purplish color on your arms and legs

Figure 25: Skin changes with increasing age.

Getting the Most out of Your Health-Care Team

When you go to see your wound specialist (or any other health-care
provider), here are some tips so you can get the most out of your visit
(see also Chapter 3).

- Phone ahead to make sure that you can easily physically access
  the clinic. For example, if you use a wheelchair, make sure that
  the clinic is wheelchair accessible.
- If you are hard-of-hearing, wear any hearing aids that you
  have and/or bring someone with you who can help you com-

municate with your wound team. If you are hard-of-hearing but do not have a hearing aid, you can purchase an inexpensive sound amplifier with headphones at a medical supply store or electronics store. With a sound amplifier, you wear headphones while the wound specialist talks into a microphone for you to hear better.

 ## What Is a Geriatric Medicine Specialist?

A geriatric medicine specialist (also known as a geriatrician) is a medical doctor who has completed specialized training in caring for older adults. You should consider asking your primary care physician for a referral to see a geriatrician if you are sixty-five years or older and have one or more of the following:

- memory problems
- urinary incontinence
- falls
- balance problems
- several medications
- feelings of being depressed
- caring for someone else and feeling stressed
- trouble doing any or all of your daily activities (grocery shopping, preparing meals, bathing yourself, managing your finances and paying the bills, and so on)

A geriatrician may or may not be a wound specialist. You can ask your wound specialist for a referral to a geriatrician if you have any of the above concerns.

- Write questions down before you go to see your wound specialist; if you wait until you are there, you may forget to discuss
  some important concerns that you had.

When Wound Healing Is Not the Goal

For some older people with many underlying serious medical illnesses,
healing the wound may not be as important as preserving dignity and
maintaining quality of life (see Chapter 31).

24
Children and Teenagers

This book is focused on caring for adults coping with wounds. Sadly, however, newborns and children can also suffer from both acute and chronic wounds. If you are caring for a child's wounds, this chapter is for you.

Most wounds in children are caused by accidents, including playground injuries, which result in more than 200,000 emergency room visits each year. Wounds in children normally heal faster than wounds in adults. However, some children suffer from slowly healing wounds, often because of diseases they were born with. The normally rapid wound-healing response of babies and children can be slowed down due to malnutrition, infection, or poor circulation. Newborns are at especially high risk for life-threatening infection because they have immature immune systems.

The skin acts like a barrier against the outside environment and protects your baby from potential dangers in the outside world, including bacteria and extreme changes in temperatures. Skin forms by 34 weeks of gestation but is not fully completed until 2 to 3 weeks after birth (no matter what the gestational age of the baby is). So if a baby is premature, the skin may not be completely formed, and your baby may be at high risk of developing infection, dehydration, and hypothermia.

Epidermolysis Bullosa

Epidermolysis bullosa (EB) includes a group of hereditary disorders of the skin that result in fragile skin that blisters with the slightest friction

> *Premature infant*: a newborn delivered before 36 weeks of
> gestation
> *Newborn*: delivery to 30 days after delivery
> *Infant*: from 30 days after delivery to 1 year of life
> *Child*: 1 year of age until 13 years of age

or trauma. Some people blister starting right at birth, while others
don't develop skin problems until late in life. The extent of blistering
in a newborn does not indicate how severe the disease is. The severity
of the disease depends on which of the four specific genetic subtypes
of EB the person has:

1. *EB simplex*: People in this category have superficial skin blisters that heal without scarring. No other parts of their body are
   affected other than their skin.
2. *Hemidesmosomal EB*: This subtype results in more extensive
   blisters than in those with EB simplex. They may also have
   problems with areas in the body that are covered with mucous
   membranes, such as the inside of their mouths. Additionally,
   they may have stomach problems or muscular dystrophy.
3. *Junctional EB*: People with this subtype typically have severe,
   nonhealing blisters on the skin as well as around the lips and
   in the mouth. They often also have severe involvement of their
   airway and breathing system.
4. *Dystrophic EB*: This is the most severe type of EB. The problem
   is with an abnormal type of collagen, which is part of the skin.
   Children with dystrophic EB have severe, extensive chronic
   blisters, resulting in scarring of the skin and contractures of
   joints. Lips, mouth, and esophagus are often affected, leading
   to impaired nutrition.

The goals of skin care of children with EB include preventing blisters from forming and also healing any existing blisters.

Preventing Blisters

Prevention of blisters is done by minimizing skin trauma. Therefore, special care is required, particularly for newborns. Newborns should have as few monitors, sticky tapes (which can tear skin), and needles as possible. Instead of tape, nonstick dressings (such as silicone dressings) or bandages can be used. For older infants and children, specially designed gear can be used to protect the areas that tend to be injured frequently, such as the knees, feet, and hands. The wound team may puncture any large blisters with a sterile needle (without cutting away the skin that was holding the fluid) and cover them with nonstick dressings to reduce pain and prevent more blisters from forming.

Treating Epidermolysis Bullosa

If and when blisters do develop, they need to be treated properly so that they heal without becoming infected. Only nonstick dressings (sometimes with a topical antibiotic) should be used, and absorbent dressings can be used for wounds that are draining. Instead of using tape, net-like elastic bandages can help to keep the dressings in place.

Debridement (surgical cleaning) of wounds is not often done for children with EB as this can lead to more blisters forming. Don't use silver-sulfadiazine cream on babies with EB, since the silver can be absorbed into their bloodstream if it is used for a long time. Some antibiotics that are taken by mouth are also anti-inflammatory, which can help to heal blisters. In addition to caring for the blisters, make sure that the child has proper nutrition and adequate pain control, and does not have any itching (as scratching can lead to more blisters).

Some nonhealing wounds in children with EB may heal well with skin substitutes—such as Apligraf or Dermagraf (see Chapter 19)—and may blister less. These skin substitutes are very expensive, and more studies are needed to see if they really do work for children with EB.

Leg Ulcers Due to Sickle Cell Disease

Sickle cell disease usually presents in the teenager or young adult, around the age of fifteen. We discuss this in more detail in Chapter 25.

Pressure Ulcers

You may think that only people who use wheelchairs or are bedbound and elderly get pressure ulcers. However, pressure ulcers can occur in one in four children in intensive care units, and in over 40 percent of people with spina bifida. Newborns and young children who are at risk most commonly get pressure sores on the back of their heads because of the large head size compared with their body size. In older children, the most common site of pressure sores is in the tailbone area.

To help prevent and treat pressure ulcers in babies and children, you need to take many of the same steps as for adults, including reducing the amount of pressure that occurs from equipment (see Part II "Pressure Sores"). Check the bed and crib carefully to make sure that tubing, other medical equipment, or toys are not lying under or on top of the child's skin. When special mattresses or cushions are used, they should be appropriate for the age and weight of the child.

Pilonidal Cysts and Sinuses

After puberty, pilonidal cysts and sinuses can form. This is a common problem and can be very frustrating because just when you think they have healed, they can occur again. Additionally, you can't see the wound yourself so you have to depend on others to look and tell you if it is better or worse. It can be embarrassing for a teenager to talk about these wounds because of where they are, and it can be difficult to keep the area clean and dry. Hair follicles near the rectum can become infected and form an abscess (a small area filled with pus). Though it can take a long time (often several months), a proper dressing such as one containing nanocrystalline silver (for example, Acticoat) may sometimes help to heal these wounds.

If the abscess remains, surgery can drain the abscess, and 60 percent of people who have this done will heal. However, for the other 40 percent, the abscess just remains an open wound after surgery, may not heal, or may heal and then open up again. Therefore, surgery is not the answer for everyone. An opinion from a colorectal surgeon can be helpful.

25
Wounds in Dark Skin

In the United States, African American and Latino populations are the fastest-growing populations over the age of eighty-five. These ethnic groups, along with Asians, Native Americans, and those of Hawaiian/ Pacific Islander descent all have high rates of certain types of chronic wounds.

The color of the skin may sometimes make it difficult for your health-care team to figure out exactly the cause of your skin problems because skin conditions can look different in darker skin than in white skin. People with dark skin are less likely to get skin cancers than people with light skin, but can still get these cancers. In addition, people with dark skin get skin cancers in different places than people with lighter skin do. These are just a couple of the issues that you and your health-care team should be aware of if you have dark skin.

Culture Clashes and the Challenging Wound

You may have a very different cultural background from your wound team. If you feel that your wound team does not respect you or your culture, or you are not able to communicate with the team because of a language barrier, do not be shy to speak up.

Many older people in North America were born elsewhere and may not speak English as their first language. If you are part of this growing group, you may have some difficulty understanding your health-care team's recommendations. It may also be difficult to make sure that *you* are understood well. It is important to have a health professional you trust. The wound team may not understand that there is a culture or language barrier.

What can you do? Express your concerns and needs. If you care for someone who does not speak English well, you can make a big difference by going to health-care appointments to aid communication between the health-care team and your loved one. This involvement can promote the best wound healing outcome. Sometimes the wound team may have the means to provide a translator at the appointment. If your loved one needs a translator, you or another team member should call before your visit and ask the receptionist in the wound office so that there will be plenty of time to arrange one.

If you still don't feel that your wound team is respectful of your culture or needs, you may be better off finding another wound team that is.

Diagnosis of Pressure Ulcers in Dark Skin

Did you know that pressure ulcers occur four times more often in dark-skinned individuals than in light-skinned individuals? People with dark skin are also more likely to develop more severe pressure ulcers. Additionally, African Americans are at high risk of developing pressure ulcers when they are admitted to a hospital.

One of the reasons pressure ulcers develop more often and become more severe in people with dark skin is probably because it is difficult to see the early warning signs of pressure ulcer development, such as slight redness. You can be the best advocate for yourself or your loved one in the clinic or hospital. Many physicians and nurses are not familiar with how to properly assess skin in dark-skinned individuals, and you can serve as a teacher for them.

If you or a loved one is dark-skinned and is at risk for developing a pressure ulcer (for example, has limited mobility or any of the other risk factors discussed in Chapter 5), speak to your wound team about how to identify early signs of pressure ulcer development so you can prevent them and treat them as quickly as possible, before they worsen.

Foot Ulcers in Non-Caucasian People with Diabetes

African Americans, Latinos, and Native Americans are at increased
risk for type 2 diabetes. African Americans in particular, are at very
high risk. More than 13 percent of African Americans over the age of
twenty have diabetes, and African Americans are almost twice as likely
to have diabetes as non-Hispanic whites. Twenty-five percent of African Americans between the ages of sixty-five and seventy-four have
diabetes, and one in four African American women over fifty-five years
of age has diabetes.

Foot ulcers are one complication of diabetes. In the United States,
dark-skinned people (especially African Americans and South Asians)
with diabetes are at higher risk for foot ulcers than light-skinned people. In the United Kingdom, South Asians with diabetes and those of
African descent do not have higher rates of foot ulceration than white
people.

African Americans with diabetes have a two to three times higher
likelihood of foot or leg amputation compared with white people with
diabetes. It is therefore important to prevent foot ulcers from happening, and treat them as early as possible.

Peripheral Arterial Disease (Poor Blood Flow)

Latinos and African Americans have a higher incidence of high blood
pressure than non-Hispanic whites. One of the results of poorly treated
high blood pressure is peripheral arterial disease: that is, poor blood
flow to the feet and legs. This results in poor wound healing, particularly in people who also have diabetes.

African Americans with poor blood flow are two to four times
more likely than white persons with poor blood flow to need an amputation of their foot or leg.

Leg Ulcers in Sickle-Cell Disease

Sickle-cell disease (SCD) is an inherited disease in which there is abnormal formation of hemoglobin (a cell in the blood which carries oxy-

gen). In people with SCD the hemoglobin carries much less oxygen than normal. Up to 70 percent of people with SCD have at least one leg ulcer in their lifetime. The risk of ulcer formation is greater if there is trauma to the leg or if the person has venous stasis. Usually, leg ulcers in people with SCD affect the inside of the lower third of the leg, with the ankle area being the most susceptible. Ulcers can also occur in young people with this disease.

Sickle-cell ulcers can be very slow to heal. The management of sickle-cell ulcers includes wound care, pain control, treatment of the anemia (which may include medications and transfusions), and control of infection. Compression with stockings or bandages can also help healing.

Leprosy

Leprosy, also known as Hansen disease, is a chronic bacterial infection. If it is not treated, it can result in permanent damage to the skin, eyes, and nerves. Up to three million people around the world are permanently disabled due to Hansen disease. The countries with the greatest number of cases are India, Brazil, and Myanmar. Some immigrants to the United States from these countries may suffer from the residual, permanent (but not contagious) results of this disease.

Damage to the nerves results in neuropathy (nerve damage). Leprosy is the most common treatable form of neuropathy in the world. As in neuropathy due to diabetes, the longest nerves in the body are often affected first: that is, nerves to the feet and lower legs. When this nerve damage occurs, affected people cannot feel any damage or trauma that occurs and may develop foot ulcers that are slow to heal. These can be treated in similar ways to foot ulcers in people with diabetes (see Part III).

Elephantiasis and Lymphedema

Elephantiasis is a disease that results in thickening of the skin and underlying tissues, especially in the legs and genitals. It occurs in some developing countries and is often caused by parasitic worms that are transmitted by mosquitoes. It is not contagious. The infection that causes elephantiasis can be treated if medications are given soon after infection. If left untreated, permanent damage can result to the lymph vessels, even after the infection itself is gone. This damage to the lymph vessels is known as lymphedema and is discussed further in Chapter 12.

Scars and Healed Wounds

Dark-skinned individuals are more likely to have noticeable scars after their wound has healed due to the melanin (pigment) in their skin. The scar can often be quite dark in color, though it may fade with time. There are some products you can buy (some require a prescription) which may fade the scar somewhat, but time is probably what will make the scar least visible. Talk to your doctor about which products would be best for you.

Keloid Scars

Dark skin also more easily forms keloids, which are raised (bumpy) scars. In fact, African Americans are ten times more likely to develop keloids than white Americans. Large amounts of scar tissue form on and around the site of your healed wound. These scars are the result of an overly aggressive healing process and can be larger than the original wound. Large keloid scars, if they are in the area of any of your joints, may affect your mobility. You need to see a dermatologist for treatment of these keloids. The dermatologist may remove the keloids surgically or may treat you by injecting steroid into the keloids. Smaller keloids can be treated using freezing therapy with liquid nitrogen. You can help prevent keloids from forming by applying some pressure, or using gel pads with silicone if you have an injury.

The Bottom Line

If you or your loved one has dark skin and has risk factors for developing a chronic wound, talk to your health-care team. Risk factors include age over sixty-five years, reduced ability to move, diabetes, sickle cell anemia, diabetes, and poor circulation. Ask your health-care team if there are certain signs you should be looking out for to prevent wounds from occurring, and to treat them early if they do occur. This can make a huge difference to you or your loved one's quality of life.

26
Wounds and Excess Weight

Mrs. A has always been overweight, but she gained a lot of additional weight when she was pregnant with each of her two children. Although she tried, she was not able to lose this weight. She became morbidly obese and developed diabetes and sleep apnea. She recently had gall bladder surgery, but the incision site did not heal well. It became infected and has caused her a lot of problems. She came to the clinic to see if there was anything we could do to help her surgical wound heal.

The Obesity Epidemic in the United States

Obesity rates in the United States are high and increasing. Sixty-seven percent of Americans are overweight, and 10 to 15 percent are considered obese. Up to one in ten Americans is morbidly obese, with a body mass index (BMI)* greater than 40. Americans spend nearly $33 billion annually in attempts to control or lose weight, whereas $100 billion is spent on obesity-related health problems.

The frequency of obesity among African American and white men is similar, but it is higher in African American women than in white women. More than 80 percent of African American women aged over forty are overweight and more than half are obese. Obesity is twice as common among women of lower socioeconomic status as among those of higher socioeconomic status. Obesity contributes to five of the ten leading causes of death and is the second most common cause of preventable death in the United States after cigarette smoking. Obesity can also complicate wound healing.

Am I Obese?

In adults, obesity is determined by body mass index, or BMI. BMI is defined as weight (in kilograms) divided by height (meters)^2. Asians and Native Americans have a lower cut-off (23 kg/m^2) for overweight. If you are very muscular with low body fat, you may have a high BMI. In children and adolescents, overweight is a BMI above the 95th percentile based on age- and sex-specific growth charts, not by using the adult BMI table.

A large waist circumference is a marker of potential health problems due to obesity (Figure 26). A waist circumference of greater than 36.3 inches (93 cm) in men or greater than 30.8 inches (79 cm) in women is a risk factor. Waist circumferences of greater than 40 inches (101.6 cm) in men or 35 inches (88.9 cm) in women are especially of concern; these individuals are at highest risk for adverse health effects.

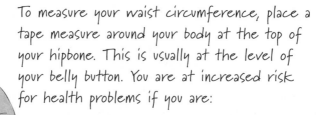

To measure your waist circumference, place a tape measure around your body at the top of your hipbone. This is usually at the level of your belly button. You are at increased risk for health problems if you are:

A man with a waist measurement greater than 40 in. (101.6 cm).

A woman with a waist measurement greater than 35 in. (88.9 cm).

Figure 26: Measuring waist circumference.

Why Does Obesity Occur?

Obesity usually results from chronic overeating *plus* not enough exercise *and perhaps* a family history of obesity. Excess caloric intake is responsible for more cases of obesity than slow metabolism alone. Family history has more of an effect on where on your body the fat sits (such as your belly or buttocks) than how overweight you actually are. More rarely, brain damage, biochemical abnormalities, and hormonal disorders (such as low thyroid hormone) can cause weight gain.

Diets high in fat and refined carbohydrates (such as white rice and sugar) promote weight gain. Diets high in fresh fruit and vegetables, fiber, and complex carbohydrates (such as whole grains) can help you to keep your weight steady or help you lose weight. A sedentary (non-active) lifestyle, with little exercise, will result in your gaining weight. Some drugs (such as steroids, lithium, some antidepressants, and sleeping pills) can increase your risk of weight gain. If you were overweight since infancy or childhood, it will be that much more difficult to lose weight later in life, so it is important to demonstrate good diet and exercise habits to children.

Pressure Ulcer Challenges When You Are Obese

We discussed pressure ulcers in detail in Part II. People who are obese have even more challenges when faced with a pressure ulcer.

You and your loved one should check your skin frequently for any skin changes or redness. Beds and wheelchairs may not fit you properly and so can put you at risk for developing a pressure ulcer. A rotating bed may help reposition you if it is difficult for health-care staff to do so frequently enough. People who weigh more than three hundred pounds generally require special equipment. This equipment can include a wide bed (so you are able to turn by yourself), a walker that can adequately support your weight, and an overhead trapeze to help you reposition yourself in bed if you cannot reposition yourself without help. These items can help you keep your muscle strength and allow you to stay independent. A physiotherapist can help you obtain such devices. Although special equipment can be helpful, it may not be enough. Be sure to communicate with your wound care team about your needs.

Some very obese people have a pannus—a large amount of abdominal skin with underlying fat that hangs over the groin and possibly the legs. The pannus must be repositioned from time to time to prevent pressure injury to the skin underneath it. You may be able to physically lift the pannus to decrease pressure to the area beneath it. If you are too weak to do this, you can try lying on your side from time to time so your loved one or health-care professional can lift the pannus away from the underlying skin surface, allowing air to flow while relieving pressure.

Fungal Infections

Fungus (a common species in humans is called *Candida*) that can infect the body thrives in a dark, moist environment, such as within skin folds. *Candida* normally lives in the mouth, gastrointestinal tract, and vagina and does not always cause infection. However, the *Candida* can overgrow and cause infection on the skin and skin folds in people who are obese. We talk more about treating fungal infections in Chapter 35.

Surgery When You Are Obese

After surgery, the surgical incision site should form a watertight seal within twenty-four hours. However, when someone is obese, the normal wound healing process can be delayed. Excess body fat increases the tension at the wound edges, making the wound prone to breaking open. There may not be enough blood supply to the fat to provide an adequate amount of oxygen and nutrients. Wound healing may also be delayed if your diet lacks essential vitamins and nutrients or if your wound is within a skin fold, where excess moisture and bacteria can build up.

If you or your loved one is obese, you should also know that something called resedation is a postoperative threat. Several hours after surgery, most of the effects of the anesthesia drugs used during surgery have left your body. Resedation occurs when the anesthetic or sedative agents that remained in the fatty tissue enter the bloodstream. The point when you're using postoperative pain medication is the time the resedation phenomenon might occur. Resedation may be life-threatening if medical attention is not received quickly enough. If you are planning for surgery, discuss this issue with your health-care providers.

Don't Give up Hope: Losing Weight for Good

The good news is that even a small amount of weight loss (as little as 5 percent of your body weight) can improve your health, allow you to live longer, and decrease your risk of getting sick. If you have obstructive sleep apnea, you will need to lose a greater amount of weight to see improvements in this condition. Studies have shown that a support system of your friends and family, as well as health-care providers, can help you lose weight and keep it off.

Strategies to help you lose weight must change how you eat and increase your physical activity. The equation of eating less and exercising more is a simple concept, but changing your lifestyle is always a challenge. You may need the support of experts and peers to make it easier to overcome. Talk to your health-care team about support for a weight-loss program. For some individuals, drugs or surgery are appropriate strategies.

Eat a balanced diet: Here are guidelines to follow:

- Low-fat, healthy diets and some calorie restriction (not less than 1000 to 1400 kcal/day)
- Substitution of some protein for carbohydrate
- Fresh fruits and vegetables as well as fiber should be substituted for refined carbohydrates and processed food
- Substitution of water for soft drinks or juices
- Fish oils or monounsaturated fats derived from plants (e.g., olive oil) reduce your risk of cardiovascular disease and diabetes.

Physical activity: Exercise increases how much energy you spend, your metabolic rate, and your ability to burn fat. Exercise also seems to

Fad Diets

Avoid diets that require atypical eating habits (such as severe calorie restriction for a long period of time—this makes your body think that it is "starving," and so the body holds onto its fat). Even if you lose weight, it will be hard to continue on these diets long term, and you will gain weight when you go back to your old eating habits.

change your appetite to more closely match your body's needs. Other benefits include improved cholesterol levels, reduced blood pressure, better fitness, and improved emotional and mental well-being. Strengthening (resistance) exercises, such as with weights, increase muscle mass. This muscle mass burns more calories than fat tissue when the body is at rest, so you burn more calories even when you are not exercising.

Most important, find a form of exercise that is interesting and enjoyable to you, whether it is walking with friends or your dog, riding your stationary bike, or swimming a few laps; you'll be more likely to stick with it.

Behavioral therapy: The goal of behavioral therapy is to improve your eating habits and physical activity level by changing the way you think about food. You are shown how to eat healthy foods (which is more effective in weight loss) rather than trying to stick with a difficult diet. You are taught how to avoid high-calorie snacks and choose satisfying but nutritional items from the menu at a restaurant. Emotional support and stress management may help you to manage the cravings that occur during any long-term weight loss program.

Drugs: Medications to help you with weight loss may be prescribed to you if your BMI is greater than 30 (or if your BMI is greater than 27 *and* there are other factors that prevent you from losing weight, such as insulin resistance). You usually only lose small amounts of weight when you use medication to promote weight loss and most of it occurs during the first six months of taking the drugs. Drugs are usually more useful for maintaining weight loss. Over-the-counter weight loss drugs are not recommended as they can be dangerous. Those containing caffeine, ephedrine, or phenylpropanolamine have side effects that can range from mild to severe.

Surgery: Surgery may be right for you if exercise, diet, and behavioral therapy have not been successful, and you are morbidly obese (BMI greater than 40) or have serious health complications. How much weight you lose depends on how severely obese you are to begin with (that is, the more obese you are, the more weight you are likely to lose from surgery). The gastric bypass is most effective. Adjustable gastric bands placed via a laparoscope, a reversible procedure, are also effective.

People do lose weight rapidly after such surgery and continue to lose weight slowly over about two years. Complications from the surgery can be significant, so it is important that an experienced surgeon perform the procedure. Some people experience chronic complications from the surgery such as vomiting and diarrhea. The large amount of weight loss results in excess skin, and many formerly obese patients require surgery to get rid of this excess flap of skin after the gastric surgery. Often, insurance may pay for your gastric surgery, but not for the surgery on this excess flap of skin. Your health-care team can discuss the appropriateness of surgery for you.

If you or your loved one undergoes this surgery, be aware that wound dehiscence (the wound opening up again after it has closed) and wound infection are common postoperative problems. Infection can be a problem because many morbidly obese people have associated medical problems (such as diabetes), which can result in slow wound healing.

Mrs. A was very upset that her wound after the gall bladder surgery was not healing. She had gone into the surgery hoping that her life would get better, but now she felt that her life was actually worse than before.

Part of the problem was that the nonhealing wound was in the middle of a heavy skin fold on her belly, so her fat was covering the wound. One of the treatment decisions that she made with her health-care team was that an abdominal binder would be used to help the wound heal (this is a snug wide band worn around the abdomen). Mrs. A decided that she would also take this opportunity to lose weight. She started walking for ten minutes a day, and eventually was walking thirty minutes a day.

She ended up losing thirty pounds over six months. She felt better, she was sleeping more soundly, and her overall mood was improved. As her wound was very deep it took a long time to heal. Mrs. A took this difficult challenge and made it an opportunity to improve her life.

27
Solutions to Stoma Struggles

Mr. N came in with a troublesome wound around his stoma. The stoma had been required after he had bowel surgery eight years earlier. Having to live with a stoma was deeply troubling for him, and the wound was making him feel worse. He became depressed and stopped working. He also was not able to change his appliance because it was so difficult for him to accept that he had to live with a stoma. When he came to the wound clinic, he would often pace the halls uncomfortably before his appointment. When we spoke with him, we could tell he really did not want to be there.

If you are coping with a stoma, you are not alone—millions of people have stomas. Skin problems relating to the stoma are extremely common.

What Are Stomas and Why Are They Necessary?

Sometimes a person has an intestinal or urinary disorder where they cannot eliminate waste in the normal way. Therefore, they need a stoma—stomas are like bags and allow for excretion of urine or feces. A stoma is a surgically created opening of the intestinal or urinary tract on the body surface. Stomas most often open via a short spout onto the surface of the abdominal wall. They may be permanent or temporary (another surgical operation is required to rejoin the bowel).

There are three types of stomas:

Ileostomy: This is an opening of the ileum (small bowel). The end or a loop of the bowel can be placed in the lower right abdomen.

Colostomy: This is an opening of the colon (large bowel). The end or a loop of the bowel is most often placed in the lower left abdomen.

Urostomy: This type of ostomy allows for urine to be excreted. It is always at the end of the bowel that may be situated in one of several places, including on the lower abdomen or on your side (between the ribs and the hips).

Some problems that can occur with the skin around your stoma are:

- Irritation (for example, bowel contents leaking onto the skin or too frequent appliance changes can irritate skin)
- Allergic reaction
- Infection
- Bleeding
- An undesired passage between the bowel and the skin (this is called a fistula)
- Pyoderma gangrenosum
- More rarely, skin cancers can occur around a stoma

Stoma Appliances

A specialist nurse will help you with selecting the most appropriate appliance and will help you adjust to living with a stoma. The pouch is made of plastic and helps to prevent leakage and protect the surrounding skin from damage. The part of the stoma that is in contact with the skin is made of sticky hydrocolloid*.

Skin Care

Cleanse the skin around the stoma with water alone, using a cotton wipe. If a cleanser is used, it should be gentle and thoroughly rinsed away after using. Avoid products with fragrance.

Shave hairy areas with an electric razor, and cover any raw areas of skin with a thin hydrocolloid before applying the stoma bag.

If you have any leaks, you can use barrier films, pastes, or powder to protect the skin.

Skin Color Changes

The skin surrounding the stoma may change color.

Brown: This usually happens after skin irritation, allergy, scar, or pyoderma gangrenosum has healed. This brown color fades over time.

Red, pink, or light purple: This may be normal, caused by the growth of new blood vessels.

White: This may be from old scars or stretch marks.

Other colors: Your skin tone may change because of urine staining.

Skin Infection

Bacteria may grow under the hydrocolloid of a stoma because the stoma is warm, humid, and contains waste products from the body. Bacteria may not always cause infection, even though they grow. Skin infection is more likely if you have diabetes, have other serious medical illnesses, or take medications that affect your immune system.

Usually, cleaning the infected skin with an antiseptic may be enough. Treatment with oral antibiotics may be necessary to get rid of a more severe infection.

Skin Irritation

If you have a stoma, you may suffer from skin irritation from time to time. Irritated skin (also called "irritant contact dermatitis") feels very sore or itchy. You may notice small red bumps and larger thick red patches, and what looks like dry, scaly skin. The irritated area may be crescent-shaped and appear below the appliance or affect the whole area in contact with it.

The main causes of skin irritation due to a stoma are:

- Constant bowel or urine leakage onto the skin
- Frequent need to change the appliance, which may strip the skin
- Friction or pressure from the appliance or clothing
- Sensitive skin or eczema
- Cleansing the skin with irritating chemicals such as certain detergents, deodorizers, or bleach

Your ostomy nurse or wound team may suggest one or more of the following treatments to help with the irritated skin:

- Modify the appliance so it fits better
- Use filler paste to make a flat surface (the bag can stick better on a flat surface)

 Your appliance may leak (resulting in bowel or urine on the skin) because of one or more of the following:

- It may be the wrong size
- It may not be on the correct site
- Skin folds due to obesity or scarring from surgery
- A great deal of sweating (which prevents sticking)
- Underlying skin rash (prevents the appliance from sticking)
- A lot of stool (for example, diarrhea) or urine

- Apply a hydrocolloid dressing (again, the bag can stick better onto this than onto irritated skin)
- Dust sucralfate onto irritated skin
- Apply roll-on antiperspirant to reduce sweat
- Use a steroid lotion as recommended by your team.

If the skin irritation has been going on for months or longer, you may start to develop very thick red skin and skin overgrowth. Your doctor may then need to use a silver nitrate stick or freezing spray to get rid of some excess skin. Very rarely, surgery to reposition the stoma may be required.

Skin Allergies

Not many people are allergic to their stoma appliance. If you do happen to be allergic to one of the above components, an allergic reaction might look like the irritated skin described above. Skin allergy may be due to components of the appliance, deodorizer, fragrance, or preservative in one of the cleansers you are using.

Your doctor may recommend that skin patch testing be performed to figure out what exactly you are allergic to.

Psoriasis

You are more likely to develop psoriasis (patches of scaly, red skin) around a stoma if you have psoriasis in other parts of your body already or if you have inflammatory bowel disease (such as Crohn's disease or ulcerative colitis). The repeated action of tearing off skin when the appliance is changed may aggravate psoriasis and make it more likely to occur.

Psoriasis may be worse just outside the stoma because sometimes the moistness under the appliance may keep the skin directly under the stoma from getting too dry. Your doctor may treat the psoriasis under or around a stoma with steroid creams (see the textbox), or other treatments such as phototherapy. You may be a candidate for other medications called biologics which treat inflammatory diseases like psoriasis, Crohn's disease, and ulcerative colitis.

Pyoderma Gangrenosum

PG can be very painful and looks like red, raised bumps or ulcers under or around your stoma. See Chapter 16 for more detail about PG.

 Rash Under Your Stoma?

Your doctor may suggest you use a steroid to treat the rash under or around your stoma. Here are some tips to using steroids (make sure you discuss any changes to your doctor's recommendation with him or her first):

- You can apply steroid lotions or steroid solutions (which are sometimes meant to be applied to the scalp, but can be useful around a stoma site if your doctor recommends it) directly to the stoma when the bag is changed. Apply the solution onto the adhesive barrier of the stoma bag and let it dry before you place the bag onto the skin. This will help avoid stinging.
- Creams and ointments are usually not practical as the appliance will not stick.
- If the steroid is only available as a cream or ointment, apply it under the hydrocolloid and stick the appliance onto this.
- Some steroids come in a paste. The paste can be placed in a skin ulcer and the appliance placed on top.

Mr. N did not initially want to spend time trying different appliances to find the right one for him. He felt that the one he was using was fine, but we disagreed. We thought it was adding pressure to the wound and actually making his life worse. In our clinic, we were able to convince him of this, and helped him learn how to change his appliance. We spent a lot of time allowing him to talk about his feelings about his stoma. He eventually accepted that he had the stoma and decided to care for it.

After he came to terms with his stoma he became much more interested in the different types of appliances that were available. The team and Mr. N worked together to find an appliance that worked for him, and after several months his wound healed.

28
Living with an Amputation

You or a loved one may have had a limb amputated because of a traumatic injury (such as a motor vehicle accident), because it was a life-saving measure (for example, when the risk of infection is high), or to improve your quality of life (as when pain in the affected limb is uncontrollable by other methods). If you have had an amputation of any kind, this chapter is for you.

Traumatic Versus Nontraumatic Amputation

One might say that every amputation is traumatic, but in medicine the term has a specific meaning. A "traumatic" amputation occurs due to an accidental injury, such as in a motor vehicle accident. A "nontraumatic" amputation is usually performed by doctors in the operating room (for example, to reduce the risk of life-threatening infection). The most common reasons for a nontraumatic amputation are:

- Diabetic foot ulcer infection or gangrene[*]
- Cancer in the bone
- Circulation problems
- Deformities of arms, legs, fingers, or toes
- Bone infection (osteomyelitis) untreatable by other methods

Whatever the reason for your amputation, it is important to take care of the skin at your amputated site. Your residual limb is at high risk of infection, especially if it sits within an airless socket (the prosthesis) all day.

Preventing skin breakdown in this area will reduce your risk of developing an infection, and will help you to have a normal, active lifestyle.

Cleaning Your Amputation Site

Cleaning your skin is important in order to keep it healthy. Clean your residual limb at the end of the day as this is the time the skin in the area is likely to be most damp. Damp skin in a socket is more likely to become irritated and infected.

Use warm water and a mild cleanser. Gently tap your skin dry. When your skin is dry, apply a moisturizer (check with your wound team first to see which moisturizer is best). We talk more about cleaning and moisturizing your skin in Chapter 35. Keeping your skin moisturized helps it to stay elastic, strong, and less likely to develop cracks (which can let in bacteria). Healthy skin is less likely to break down or form ulcers, even with the high pressure that can be placed on it by your prosthesis.

Taking Care of Your Prosthesis

The prosthetic socket can become too moist and develop into a breeding ground for bacteria and fungus if it is not cleaned properly and regularly. It is important to wash the prosthetic socket daily, preferably at the end of the day. Sockets with valves need special attention since microorganisms can become trapped in the valves. Be sure to remove any valves and wash and rinse them. Wash the socket itself thoroughly using warm water and mild soap. Rinse the soap off *completely* and pat the socket and valves dry with a towel. You can then leave them out to dry overnight. Make sure before you place the prosthesis on again that the socket is dry, unless your prosthetist has advised otherwise. Too much moisture can irritate your skin.

Taking Care of Your Prosthetic Sock, Sheath, and Insert

The prosthetic sock and sheath absorb your sweat and any bacteria and fungus from your skin. To get rid of these microorganisms, you need to clean your sock and sheath daily, and change your socks at least once during the day. Use a mild detergent to wash both the sock and sheath (hand wash or use the delicate cycle), rinse them well, gently squeeze the water out, and hang them up or lay flat to dry. You can towel dry your insert. Your sheath may need up to two days to dry fully. A tennis ball or sock-drying form can be used to keep your sock's shape while it dries. Make sure the sock is dry before you wear it again. Talk to your prosthetist if you sweat a lot and need a powder to use in your sock to help keep your skin from getting too wet.

Skin Allergies, Infection, and Irritation Among Amputees

Many of the skin problems that occur in people with amputations are common in people without amputations also (see Chapter 35). Even if you take excellent care of your skin and prosthetic equipment, you may still develop skin irritation, allergies, or infections. If you notice any changes in your skin, call your prosthetist, doctor, or wound team immediately.

29
The Wounds of War

While serving in the military in Iraq, Mr. M lost his leg when a roadside bomb exploded. He was eventually fit for a prosthetic leg. Mr. M is active, independent, and lives a normal life with the prosthesis. Although he can no longer work in active combat duty, he volunteers with the Disabled Veterans Associations to help others.

Thanks to improved medical care, 90 percent of soldiers who are injured in the conflicts in Iraq and Afghanistan survive. However, a new generation of physically and emotionally wounded veterans is now returning home. Many come home having lost an arm or leg.

Amputations and Prostheses

After loss of an arm or leg, prostheses can be fitted. As a result of the amputations in the Iraq War, there have been advances in prosthetics, such as anatomic socket designs and silicone gel liners. A new innovation is the "biohybrid," which treats the prosthesis as if it is part of the person's body. The biohybrid uses implantable sensors and regenerated tissue, so there can be direct nerve control of the artificial limb. An ankle-foot prosthesis that allows for a normal human gait has already been developed and is in the testing phases. We talk further about prostheses in Chapter 28.

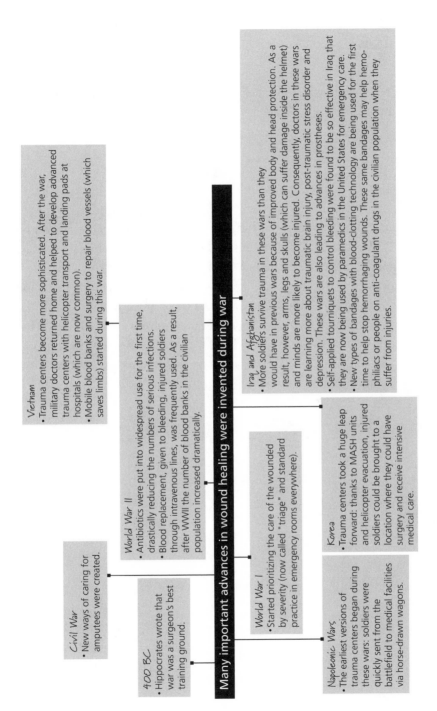

Figure 27: Advances in medical care that have occurred in wartime.

Paralysis

Some soldiers are returning from war with spinal cord injuries and
have to grapple with the challenges of paralysis. We talk extensively
about paralysis and spinal cord injury in Chapter 22.

Medical Advances

Throughout history, the experiences of doctors in wartime have led to
advances in civilian medical care (Figure 27). The tragedies of war are
immense, but the potential for the advancement in medicine can be
greatly beneficial to our veterans and our society as a whole.

Regenerative medicine is a field that has grown out of the latest
advances from the Iraq and Afghanistan wars. Regenerative medicine
is still mostly in the research phase, but its ultimate goal is to allow the
body to regenerate living tissue, rather than rely on artificial parts. One
example is the skin-cell gun, which would allow for burn victims to
have skin stem cells sprayed directly on their wounds. Eventually, it is
hoped, these stem cells would grow into skin.

30
Wounds and Cancer

Up to one in ten people with cancer develop nonhealing wounds. A wound may appear at the site of the cancer (for example, on the breast in some people with late-stage breast cancer) or at a location far away from the cancer. The cancer can be present in the wound itself, or a person with cancer can develop wounds for other reasons. Some cancers may ulcerate as they outgrow their blood supply.

In Chapter 17, we discussed skin cancers that develop in wounds. In this chapter, we look at other kinds of wounds associated with cancer.

Why Wounds Occur in People with Cancer

Certain cancers are more likely to cause nonhealing wounds. Cancers that develop into wounds are usually breast cancers, but they can also occur from cancer of the head, neck, chest, abdomen, kidney, lung, ovary, colon, and penis as well as from leukemia, lymphoma, and melanoma.

When a cell becomes cancerous, it begins to rob the normal surrounding tissues of oxygen and nutrients. Cancer cells produce chemicals that encourage blood vessels to grow into the tumor (Figure 28). This provides the tumor with a rich blood supply that helps feed the tumor. When this tumor grows and takes over the skin cells, the end result is a wound made up of cancer cells that do not have the ability to heal like normal cells do. These wounds bleed easily because they have a lot of blood vessels and do not clot well.

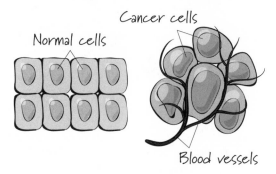

Figure 28: Cancer cells produce chemicals that encourage blood vessels to grow into the tumor.

Characteristics of Malignant Wounds

Malignant wounds tend to have a large amount of necrotic (dead) tissue. Necrotic tissue* is a comfortable home for bacteria: it is usually moist and bacteria can eat the dying tissue. These ideal living conditions allow bacteria to multiply quickly. It is this overgrowth of bacteria which can cause these wounds to have a foul odor.

Chemotherapy and Radiation

Treatment for cancer usually includes chemotherapy and/or radiation.

Chemotherapy

As a side effect, chemotherapy drugs, because they target fast-growing cancer cells, can also reduce infection-fighting cells (which are also fast growing). Therefore, the immune system is not as strong as usual. Other adverse effects of chemotherapy include gastrointestinal disturbances and sores in the mouth (or mucous membranes). Gastrointestinal disturbances, such as chronic diarrhea, can lead to irritated or chafed skin, which can make a person more likely to develop infections and wounds. Mouth sores may develop in someone with a blunted immune system. Make sure to tell your wound team if you have received chemotherapy and suffered from these or other adverse effects.

Wounds can also develop if chemotherapy drugs leak into the healthy tissues. Some chemotherapy drugs damage nerves and skin, thus causing pain or inflammation in the skin and underlying tissues.

Radiation Therapy

Radiation-induced skin damage can appear in different ways. You or your loved one may experience:

- Mild redness and swelling, similar to a sunburn
- Itching, peeling, and flaking skin
- Blisters
- Damage to hair follicles and sweat glands
- Skin ulcers and dead tissue

The exposed skin is also more prone to skin cancers in the future.

Other Effects of Chemotherapy and Radiation

Chemotherapy and radiation can alter your sense of taste. For example, some chemotherapeutic drugs will cause a metallic taste in the mouth. The disturbances along the digestive track commonly caused by chemotherapy and radiation are nausea, vomiting, and ulcerations throughout the GI system. This can make it more difficult to eat and make it more difficult for your body to manage food.

Since nutrition is key for wound healing, poor appetite and a lack of food tolerance can be a real problem. Dealing with a life-threatening illness can also cause depression and anxiety. This, along with not eating enough to sustain you, makes coping even more of a challenge.

Managing a Cancerous Wound

Though chemotherapy and radiation treatments can cause wounds, they can reduce the size of some cancerous wounds. The smaller wound may become more manageable in terms of drainage, odor, and bleeding. However, these therapies have important side effects: chemotherapy and radiation may also cause the skin around the wound to become irritated, which may lead to further wound development.

Treatment of the underlying cancer is the most important aspect to managing the wound. Local wound care should be performed as described in Part VII. You should discuss your goals of care with your wound team, as in some instances quality of life and minimizing odor and pain are more important than wound healing (see Chapter 31).

31
Wounds in the Dying
When Comfort Comes First

Mrs. S is a seventy-nine-year-old woman with advanced Alzheimer's dementia and pressure ulcers. She is lovingly cared for at home by her husband and daughter, with the help of a nurse for two hours a day. Mrs. S is not able to turn by herself, and when she is turned by her family or nurses, she groans and is clearly in pain. Her husband arranges for an ambulance to bring her to our clinic every two months. He realizes that his wife's medical problems cannot be cured, and aggressive treatment is only making her miserable. He decides that he wants to focus on keeping her comfortable instead.

If you or a loved one has a wound that cannot heal for any reason, or is at the end of life, the goals of wound treatment should be based on symptom control and comfort, rather than only on wound healing. It is very important that the focus of care is to make you as comfortable and pain-free as possible. You and your loved one should talk to your wound team to ensure that you are all on the same page regarding goals of care and that you understand the correct procedure for dressing changes. Controlling pain, drainage, and odor, minimizing infection, and using appropriate dressings are all important in enhancing dignity and quality of life.

Establishing Goals of Care in Wound Management

Aggressive treatment plans to heal wounds can be painful and emotionally distressing. This is not the best option when the wound cannot
heal for some reason (such as severe irreversible circulation problems)
or if a person has a life-threatening illness (such as end-stage dementia
or end-stage cancer). In these cases, wound care should be gentle and
as pain-free as possible.

Be sure to discuss the goals of care for yourself or a loved one with
your wound care team, so that all of you understand what the goals
are. The most important goals of the wound care team in these situations are to decrease the frequency of dressing changes, use pain-free
dressings, control wound odor, and reduce the risk of infection. Your
wound team can help you make some of these care plan decisions and
tell you what the likelihood of wound healing may be.

Modifying Wound Care in Later Life

Wound Debridement

Wound debridement and cleaning can reduce the amount of dead tissue and bacteria in a wound. Several options are available, including
use of special gels or creams to do the work. Debridement can be painful and in some cases can increase the risk of infection. In wounds that
cannot heal, or in people at the end of life, debridement may be an
unnecessarily painful procedure.

The decision to use a specific method of debridement depends on
several factors, such as:

- Cause of the wound
- The wishes of you and your family
- Other medical illnesses
- Likelihood that the wound will heal
- Risk for bleeding and pain
- Goals of care

Treating Infection

An infection in a wound can be treated with antibiotics applied topically to the wound, given by mouth, or administered through an intravenous line. Usually, giving the antibiotics by mouth or intravenously is most effective; however, a person who is dying may not be able to swallow or may have limited vein access, which makes these methods unnecessarily aggressive and painful. Talk to your wound team and decide on an approach for treating infection in advance.

Controlling Pain

Pain is an important issue in nonhealing wounds. Even if your loved one is not able to tell you how much pain they are in because they have problems verbally communicating, your health-care team can use certain pain assessment tools to help determine a person's level of pain.

Talk to your wound team about the best ways to manage pain effectively: this can be done by using special dressings, reducing the frequency of dressing changes, and giving pain medications before dressing changes are performed. In addition, topical anesthetic creams ("freezing") may reduce the amount of pain experienced by the patient during dressing changes and throughout the day. Applying creams that can freeze the skin thirty to sixty minutes before debridement or dressing changes can be effective in reducing the pain associated with these procedures. It may also be helpful for you to have control over how fast a dressing is removed, and removing the dressing yourself may help. Another helpful technique is asking the wound care specialist to talk you through each step of your dressing change, as you may feel better prepared if you know what is going to happen next. Complementary therapies, such as massage, visualization, and aromatherapy, may also help with pain control.

Choosing Dressings

Some nonhealing wounds (particularly those caused by cancer) can bleed quite a lot. Dressings made of soft silicone or petroleum jelly will not stick to the wound. Nonstick dressings reduce trauma to the wound, pain, and bleeding.

There are several dressings available that can help manage your symptoms such as pain and odor. We list many of these options in "Wound Cleansers and Dressings" in the back of the book.

CONTROLLING DRAINAGE

Controlling drainage is one of the primary goals of managing non-healing wounds. Several dressing options are available, including calcium alginate, foam, and hydrofiber dressings, which can absorb large amounts of drainage. Some dressings such as calcium alginate, Spongostan, and Oxycel reduce bleeding because they help the blood to clot. Some of these absorbent dressings (such as calcium alginate) should be used only if there is a lot of drainage because otherwise they can stick to the wound and cause damage when they are removed.

CONTROLLING ODOR

Wound odor can be reduced by using special odor-controlling dressings such as those that contain charcoal (for example, CarboFlex or Actisorb Plus) or placing a small plate of an odor absorber (such as kitty litter, charcoal, or coffee grounds) in the room. Frequent dressing changes (if they don't cause pain or discomfort) can also aid in odor control. In addition, the use of topical antibiotics may reduce bacterial load and reduce odor. The topical application of metronidazole (Metrogel) and the use of maltodextrin powder or gel can also decrease odor in some wounds.

We asked Mr. S what he thought was causing his wife the most pain and distress. He felt that changing her dressings daily was too much because she screamed whenever anyone touched her dressings. Additionally, she was also very uncomfortable being moved or turned. Furthermore, bringing her to clinic every two months was difficult, as he had to arrange for transport and she needed to be carried onto a stretcher into the ambulance and travel several miles.

We talked to Mr. S for a long time about his wishes, since he held durable power of attorney for his wife. He understood that without regular turning, her wound was unlikely to heal. Mrs. S's nutrition was so poor that it was also interfering with healing. We suggested that Mrs. S start on absorbent dressings that only needed changing three times a week, and we told Mr. S to turn her only if she was not having pain. We also did not make any more regular appointments for her; instead, we told Mr. S to call us if he had any concerns and that we were happy to see his wife at any time. Four months later, Mr. S called to tell us that Mrs. S had passed away. He was of course very upset, but was relieved that for the last few months of her life, Mrs. S had been comfortable and pain free.

PART NINE

Beyond the Wound

32
Eating Well
The Healing Potential of Food

Mrs. W is a ninety-year-old widow who lives alone with her cat, whom she loves very much. Mrs. W does not have children and her sister recently died. After a knee replacement surgery, while still in the hospital, she developed a pressure ulcer on her back. This ulcer was not healing, even after several months.

When she came to our wound clinic, she admitted that she has been finding it difficult to get out of the house to do her grocery shopping and consequently she ate mostly tea and toast. She told us that she refused to go into long-term care because she does not want to give up her cat.

Proper nutrition is crucial for the body to heal itself effectively. After surgery, if your surgical wound heals but you have poor nutrition, your wound may split open. After any type of surgery, the body quickly uses up its stores of nutrients, especially if you have a wound that is draining a great deal. Eating well also helps maintain a healthy immune system which can be important for fighting infection. It is important for you and your health-care team to develop a plan to make sure your diet, nutrient, and water intake is sufficient.

Malnutrition is common among people with chronic wounds. One out of three people admitted to surgical wards in hospitals are malnourished, and almost two out of three people admitted to non-surgical wards are malnourished. How well you are nourished affects whether you will develop a wound, how well you can heal, and even how long you may need to be in the hospital after an illness.

The problem gets even worse the older we get: a whopping three out of four people over sixty-five years of age who are admitted to the hospital are malnourished.

What does "malnourished" mean? A person is considered "malnourished" if he or she is not eating the right foods to supply the body with the nutrients it needs. Our bodies break down our food into building blocks (nutrients, sugars, fats, carbohydrates). These building blocks are then circulated through our bodies and brought to areas where they are needed. When there are not enough building blocks over a long period of time, the body sometimes will start com-

 Body Weight: When to Be Concerned

Checking your weight weekly can help monitor whether you are gaining or losing weight.

If you or your loved ones experience any of the following changes *within six to twelve months,* you need to seek help from your medical team and/or dietician *immediately,* because they indicate severe (and possibly life-threatening) weight conditions:

1. Loss of 5 percent of your normal body weight
2. Weight less than 90 percent of ideal body weight
3. Weight gain or loss of ten pounds or more
4. Obesity
5. Weight gain of 20 percent above your normal body weight

pensating by breaking down its own tissues, putting the body into a nutritional deficit. This deficit means the body is malnourished.

Because nutrition is so important, your wound team may consult a dietician to speak with you.

What Should You Be Eating?

Proper nutrition does not just mean that you eat enough. It is also important to eat the right *types* of food. Before making changes to your diet, however, you should speak with your doctor and/or a registered dietician to ensure that these changes are right for you. Let's go over the most important nutrients necessary to prevent wounds and heal any that you have that are slow to heal.

Protein

Skin is made mostly of protein, and protein is crucial for wounds to heal properly. The body needs protein to form a substance called collagen*, which is required for the healing process. If you don't take in enough protein, collagen formation is reduced or delayed and the healing process slows.

A healthy adult usually needs about 0.8 g/kg per day of protein. This means eating one or two 3-ounce servings of protein each day in the form of meat, milk, cheese, or eggs. Other ways to increase your protein intake are to use vegetable protein powder (sprinkled into food and drinks), protein shakes, and protein bars.

If you have been ill recently and lost a lot of weight, you may need to double the normal recommended dietary amount of protein in order to heal properly. As much as half of your lost weight may have to be regained before you can start to heal. If you have a wound that drains a lot of fluid, this drainage alone could be depleting you of up to 100 grams of protein per day. If you lack protein reserves, you will heal slowly, if at all, and if you are borderline malnourished, you can easily become malnourished if your wound continues to drain heavily.

Albumin is one of the most important types of protein in your body. Your wound care team may send you for blood work to check the level of albumin in your blood. Albumin is important for wound healing because:

- If albumin levels are low, the body lacks an important building block for repairing any damage to the skin.
- Studies of malnourished patients show that they have lower levels of albumin, which results in less oxygen getting into the blood and tissues, and, in turn, a reduction in the ability to kill bacteria. If this happens, you may be at higher risk of getting an infection.
- Albumin prevents fluid from leaking out of blood vessels into nearby tissues. If albumin levels fall very low, the fluid leaks out and you could develop edema (fluid leakage into tissues), which slows wound healing. If severe edema occurs, you could also develop low blood pressure as fluid leaks out of the bloodstream. If blood pressure falls to the point where there is not enough blood getting to the wound, healing may slow or may stop completely.

Other Nutrients Important for Wound Healing

In addition to protein, the body needs some fat and carbohydrates to make collagen. Vitamins A, B-complex, C, and E and the minerals iron, copper, zinc, and calcium are also important in the healing process. If you don't take in enough zinc, the top layer of skin doesn't form as quickly as it normally would, and the collagen formed is weaker, meaning that healing skin is not as strong as it should be. It is important to know the correct doses of vitamins and minerals to take, however, as "too much of a good thing" can be toxic. Be sure to discuss any supplements that you take with your health-care provider.

Are You Drinking Enough Water?

Three out of four Americans are chronically dehydrated. This problem is particularly common in persons over the age of seventy-five years and can cause severe problems such as poor wound healing, confusion, and falls. Even mild dehydration will slow down your metabolism and reduce how fast and how well your wound heals. You probably need about six glasses of water a day, but speak to your dietician and health-care team to be clear on what exactly you need to heal optimally.

Risk Factors for Poor Nutrition

There are many reasons why poor nutrition may occur. To see if you or your loved one is at risk, answer the following questions:

1. Do you have any physical limitations (the ability to eat and access food)?
   - Are you able to chew?
   - Are you able to swallow?
   - Can you keep food down or do you gag or vomit?
   - Can you access the food in your home (for example, can you get to the refrigerator)? Are you able to prepare a meal?
   - Do you suffer from paresis or paralysis (for example, after stroke)?
   - Have you had recent major surgery?
2. Do you have emotional and mental issues that may affect eating?
   - Are you depressed or do you not feel like eating?
   - Do you or your loved one have memory problems and forget to eat?
3. Do you suffer from any medical conditions?
   - Many medical conditions interfere with the body's ability to absorb nutrition.
   - Do you have high blood sugar or diabetes?
   - Do you have a medical condition (such as emphysema) that results in low oxygen in your blood?
   - Do you have kidney disease?
   - Have you experienced severe trauma (such as head injury)?
   - Have you had recent chemotherapy or radiation therapy?

- Do you have neurologic, cardiac, or thyroid problems?
- Do you have a family history of diabetes or heart disease?
- Do you have any draining wounds or fistulas?
- Do you have gastrointestinal problems (such as diarrhea or constipation)?
- Do you have mouth, tooth, or denture problems?

4. Are you taking any medications or do you drink alcohol? Are you on a special diet?
    - Are you on or have you recently been on a fad diet (such as eating only one type of food, or eliminating foods with good nutritional value)?
    - Have you used steroids, diuretics, or antacids?
    - Do you have excessive alcohol intake (that is, more than two drinks per day)?
    - Are you on a vegetarian diet that may not be providing enough protein?
    - Have you recently been on a liquid diet or had nothing by mouth for more than three days?

5. What lifestyle factors could affect your nutrition?
    - Do you have a home, and do you feel safe there?
    - Are you able to financially afford to eat properly?
    - Do you have support systems, like family or friends, to help provide food for you?
    - Do you have access to a stove and a refrigerator, and can you use them safely?

If you answered "yes" to any of the questions under numbers 1–4, and "no" to any of the questions under number 5 ("lifestyle factors"), you may be at risk of being malnourished. Speak to your wound team, and they may be able to help.

I Am Overweight—Can I Still Be Malnourished?

Just because someone is overweight does not mean he or she has good nutrition; in fact, it probably means just the opposite. If you have been eating too much of the wrong types of food (for example, fat that makes you overweight, but not enough protein), you'll be even less likely to eat the foods that will help you heal.

If you are obese, you may have an additional problem that makes wound healing even slower: adipose tissue (fat) does not have a good blood supply. As the amount of adipose tissue increases, blood flow to the skin decreases. This reduces the amount of oxygen and nutrients reaching the wound area, which slows healing and increases the risk of a new wound forming. Additionally, if there are a lot of folds in your skin due to adipose tissue, moisture and fungal infections may form, and you will be more likely to develop wounds in these areas.

If you are concerned that you may be overweight, discuss it with your wound team. They can refer you to a dietician who will be able to help (and see Chapter 26).

The Take-Home Message

It can be difficult to eat the proper nutrients needed to heal your wound. Talk to your wound team, which can go over your options for optimizing your nutritional status and improving your overall health. Changing eating habits can be difficult, but eating well is essential not only for wound healing but also for your general well-being.

We sent Mrs. W to get some blood work, which showed that she was dehydrated and deficient in iron. She was admitted to the hospital for a couple of days in order to receive some IV fluids.

During that time we were able to find a long-term care facility that allowed cats. In the facility, she was able to eat communal meals (she liked the company) and was also started on some vitamins and an iron supplement to help her nutritional state.

Several months after her move, her wound finally started to heal. Mrs. W is now able to enjoy her life (and time with her cat) because she feels comfortable and has the help she needs.

33
Exercise for Wound Healing

You've heard it before: exercise is good for you. It helps you lose weight, stay flexible, keeps you strong, and reduces the risk of many health problems such as diabetes and heart disease. What you may not have heard before is that exercise also probably helps your wounds heal faster.

One study found that regular exercise may speed up wound-healing by as much as 25 percent. In this study, the participants began with ten minutes of warm-up floor exercises and stretching, followed by thirty minutes of pedaling on a stationary bike. After that, participants either jogged or walked briskly on a treadmill for fifteen minutes, followed by about fifteen minutes of strength training. All sessions ended with five minutes of cool-down exercises. At the end of the study, the researchers found that skin wounds healed an average of ten days faster in the people who exercised.

Another study compared wound-healing rates between older adults caring for a loved one with Alzheimer's disease to rates of older adults who weren't caregivers. Wounds among caregivers took about 20 percent longer to completely heal than the noncaregivers' wounds. Caregivers may take longer to heal because of the amount of emotional and physical stress they are under, and also because they are probably not taking care of themselves (by eating well and exercising) as well as they are taking care of their loved one.

No matter what type of wound you may have, there is most likely some form of exercise that will help you heal.

Exercise for People with Foot Ulcers and Diabetes

Exercise helps to improve your blood flow, especially if you have dia-betes. Exercise works in a similar way to insulin: it moves sugar from the blood into the muscles, and this lower blood sugar results in more endurance and less fatigue.

If you have a foot ulcer, or have had a previous foot ulcer, you are at risk for developing a new or worsening wound if you do not wear the correct footwear during exercise, or do incorrect exercises. Your risk of exercising needs to be weighed against the risks of not exercising. It is important that you speak with your wound team about what they recommend for you. They may recommend specific types of exercise and special footwear in order to reduce any risks.

Exercise and Pressure Ulcers

Even though bed rest is sometimes prescribed, no good studies have ever proven that bed rest is effective for the treatment of pressure ul-cers. In fact it is just the opposite: many studies have shown that bed rest has many negative effects, including increasing depression, wors-ening immobility, and worsening pressure ulcers. Therefore, getting out of bed, changing position, and exercising are all important in the healing of pressure ulcers, as well as for your mental and emotional health.

If you are a caregiver for a person with limited mobility (such as someone with severe dementia or Parkinson's disease), a phys-iotherapist or occupational therapist can show you some simple movements you can do with your loved one to help improve their body function and blood flow, and reduce their risk of pressure ul-cers. These therapists can come to your home to show you these exercises, and can also help you and your loved one with position-ing and transfers that limit the amount of friction and shear. Talk to your wound team about a referral to physiotherapy or occupational therapy.

Exercise for People with Limited Mobility

Exercise is a healthy habit for people who use wheelchairs, as it can improve heart health, help you maintain your best possible weight, and improve your overall ability to function independently. A recent study found that people with spinal cord injuries who have healthy habits (including good nutrition, a healthy body weight, exercise, strong mental and emotional health, no use of tobacco, recreational drugs, or alcohol) are much less likely to develop a pressure ulcer five or more years after their injury than people whose lifestyle habits are not as healthy.

Exercise can be difficult for people with severely limited mobility, such as a high spinal cord injury, but can still be done. A qualified care attendant or therapist can assist you. Correctly performed exercises can help you avoid contractures (when joints become permanently inflexible) and help to maintain fitness. Range-of-motion exercise can be particularly useful. Some people with tetraplegia (quadriplegia) may be able to exercise unaided. For example, former skiing champion Jill Kinmont Boothe, who is tetraplegic, performs a daily seated aerobic exercise routine. Some people with tetraplegia can perform specific muscle-strengthening exercises. The key to exercise if you have tetraplegia is to find exercises that do not require holding or grasping.

Perhaps more important than the physical benefits of exercise is the psychological benefit. It helps you feel better about yourself and can help you move forward emotionally after your injury.

Exercise in Venous Ulcers and Lymphedema

Although sitting with your legs down or standing still for long periods of time can worsen wounds due to venous stasis or lymphedema, exercise (in addition to compression recommended by your wound team) can improve wound healing. Exercise strengthens and moves your calf muscles, which results in improved blood flow return up your legs toward the heart.

Walking can be an excellent form of exercise for people with leg swelling due to venous stasis or lymphedema. In one study, raised-leg exercises done for twenty minutes, three times a day, were very effective for reducing leg swelling.

Exercise and Peripheral Arterial Disease

More than twenty studies have shown that exercise is very effective for treating peripheral arterial disease (poor blood flow). When you exercise, blood flow is increased up to ten times the amount as when you are resting. Regular exercise may help train muscles to work more efficiently with less blood and also increases new blood vessel formation. Exercise has been shown to improve the length of time you are able to walk better than angioplasty (a "balloon" to open up blockages in your blood vessels) or blood thinners.

Many people with peripheral arterial disease suffer from calf pain when they walk a certain distance. Unfortunately, this can be a catch-22 because many people reduce the amount they walk so they won't have the calf pain. However, there is good news. Exercise can actually help to reduce this calf pain over time. Regular walking results in improvements of 80 to 234 percent in most people with calf pain due to poor blood flow. A daily walking program of a total of forty-five to sixty minutes is recommended; or, you should walk until the calf pain occurs, rest until the pain is reduced, then start to walk again. You will gain the most if each exercise session lasts at least thirty minutes, if you perform the exercises at least three times per week, when you walk until you almost cannot endure the pain, and when you keep up the program for at least six months.

How Should I Start an Exercise Program?

Before starting any type of exercise program, consult your doctor. If you have not exercised in a while, you will need to start slowly so you do not cause too much stress to your heart, lungs, muscles, and joints. If your wound team says that you can exercise, your routines should include aerobic activity, strength training, and flexibility exercises. You should exercise slowly and regularly.

Walking is often the best form of exercise. If you are not able to walk, a stationary exercise bicycle may be a good option. Start slow—

even fifteen minutes three times a week is a good start. You can then increase your sessions by five minutes every week. You should not increase your exercise by more than 10 percent from one week to the next. For example, if you walk twenty minutes one week, you should only walk twenty-two minutes the next week. If you do not recover from an exercise routine in twenty-four to thirty-six hours, talk to your doctor.

Swimming is not a good exercise option if you have an open wound. Water that is not sterile can slow wound healing by making the skin around the wound soaking wet and prone to getting worse and developing infection. The chlorine in swimming pools can irritate wounds. Fresh water ponds and the ocean contain microorganisms that can increase your risk of wound infection.

If you do not want to exercise or can only participate in limited exercise, you can blend exercise into life activities. For example, you could park in a spot farther from a store, take the stairs instead of an elevator or escalator, and do activities like household chores or gardening. It is important to figure out how to incorporate regular exercise into your life. If you treat exercise like an appointment, you are more likely to stick to a routine. It is important to keep in mind that whatever exercise you choose to do, it should feel good to you. Health professionals such as physiotherapists and occupational therapists can help design an exercise routine that is right for you.

As with any other activity that you undertake, make exercising safe. Check with a health-care professional who is trained in your particular condition (for example, spinal cord injury) before starting any type of exercise. While you are exercising, be sure to avoid friction that could irritate or scrape your skin, and be sure to wear the proper footwear.

Most important . . . have fun!

34
Pain
The Burden of Suffering

Mrs. V is a forty-eight-year-old lady with diabetes and a foot ulcer.
She doesn't have any pain in the ulcer itself, but for a long time has
had burning, numbness, and tingling in her feet. Sometimes at night
these symptoms get so bad that she has to take the bedcovers off her feet,
because they aggravate the pain.

Pain in a slow-to-heal wound can be distressing. The pain can decrease your ability to function and do things that you normally would
do, such as go to work or spend time with friends. Pain can affect you
not only physically, but also emotionally and mentally. The mental and
emotional aspects of pain and wound healing are discussed further in
Chapter 36. In this chapter, we will discuss the physical pain itself, and
what you can do to help prevent and manage it.

What Is the Purpose of Pain?

Pain has an important job—it indicates to the body that something is
wrong. For example, pain or any change in pain can indicate that a
wound is infected or otherwise getting worse.

We often praise people for being stoic in the face of pain—but
putting up with it without telling your health professional can be

dangerous. Pain (or even the fear of pain) also can impair healing by slowing down the immune response to an infection. This is one reason to talk to your wound team about any pain you are having instead of "grinning and bearing it."

Know Your Pain

It is important that you tell your wound team about any wound pain that you may be having, even if they do not ask you first . . . remember, they cannot read your mind (Figure 29). Pain is sometimes overlooked by health professionals because no simple diagnostic test exists to measure it.

 Talking About Pain with Your Wound Team

It is crucial to tell your wound team the exact details of your pain. However, the specifics can be really hard to remember—unless you write them down. This allows your pain to be better managed because different types of pain require different types of treatments. You may find it useful to keep a pain diary in which you write down the times you have pain, when it gets worse, what exactly it feels like, and so on. Take this pain diary in with you when you go to see your wound team.

Once you start treatment for the pain, write notes in your pain diary about how much medication you are taking and whether it is helping. In this way, the pain diary can be very helpful after you start treatment, by demonstrating whether the treatment is reducing the pain.

It is important for your wound team to know
how your pain affects your life.

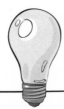

The first step to improving your pain:
remember or write down the answers to these questions
(and take them to your wound team):

- Location: in what part of the body does the pain occur? Does it spread anywhere else?

- Onset: when does the pain start? (for example, while cleaning the wound, while doing dressing changes, or something else)

- Duration: how long does the pain last?

- Intensity: how bad is the pain? Often your wound team will ask, "On a scale of 1 to 10, with 10 being the worst pain you have ever had, how bad does the pain get?"

- Quality: what does the pain feel like? For example, is it a sharp, knife-like pain? Or is it a dull ache?

- Impact: Are you able to get out of bed in the morning? Get dressed? Go to work? Take care of your kids/parent and/or spouse?

Figure 29: Your wound team needs to know details about your pain.

What Your Wound Team Can Do to Minimize Your Pain

As with other aspects of your wound care, you need to work with your wound team to help minimize your pain. Discuss with them what does and doesn't work for you. Pain specialists and pain clinics can be very helpful if your own wound team is not able to treat your pain. However, these specialists are not always available, and it can take a long time to get in to see one.

Removing the cause of the wound is probably the best way to manage the pain and can eliminate whatever is causing the pain in the first place: for example, reducing pressure in pressure ulcers. Likewise, initiating strategies to increase arterial flow in ischemic ulcers may help reduce related chronic wound pain, and treating wound infection can help reduce pain by reducing any inflammation caused by bacteria.

Types of Wound Pain

There are different types of wound pain. Your pain diary can help your wound team figure out which type or types of pain you have. Specific strategies and medications help with each type.

1. *Persistent pain:* This type of pain is constant. Medications may be necessary to treat this type of pain, but you might first want to try strategies that do not involve medications (see below, "Managing Your Pain Without Medications").
2. *Occasional procedure pain:* This type of pain occurs with certain procedures, such as when your wound team cleans or debrides your wound. Use of local anesthesia (that is, "freezing" the painful area with a cream or tiny needle) or taking a medication by mouth thirty to forty-five minutes before the procedure can help reduce this pain. Many people also find that having your wound care specialist explain exactly what he or she is about to do can help with the pain.
3. *Regular procedure pain:* This type of pain occurs regularly and predictably, such as when your wound dressings are changed.

Some things that can help are using nonstick dressings, soaking your dressings before removing them, and removing the dressings yourself instead of having the nurse do it. Discuss these options with your wound team.

Managing Your Pain Without Medications

Research shows that people who educate themselves about what could be causing their pain actually experience improvement in their pain. Participating in therapeutic exercise programs can also improve pain, especially persistent pain. Other things that can help improve wound pain include cold therapy, warmth therapy, transcutaneous electrical nerve stimulation, and acupuncture. All of these modalities result in the release of natural opioids (painkillers) in your body without you having to take medications.

Relaxation techniques, biofeedback, or hypnosis also may be useful. Physical therapy and occupational therapy have been shown to reduce pain, and can include the use of braces or splints, changes in biomechanics, and exercise. Nerve blocks (which are performed by anesthesiologists) and tumor site radiation (for those with cancer pain) also can be helpful in certain circumstances. Some people find pain relief through naturopathy or spiritual healing.

Dressing removal is usually when most people with chronic wounds experience the worst pain. Dried-out or sticky dressings are most likely to cause pain during dressing changes. Gauze dressings are also likely to cause pain. Applying and removing vacuum therapy can also cause pain in some people. Products designed to be nonstick (also called "nonadherent") can help to reduce pain during dressing changes. Newer products such as soft silicone dressings and gels are least likely to cause pain. Avoid dressings or creams that commonly cause allergic reactions—these reactions can result in painful inflammation and itching. Look at the label and avoid the following ingredients: neomycin, bacitracin, lanolin, and fragrance.

Nondrug interventions can also help during procedural pain, such as when your wound team is cleaning or debriding your wound. Proper positioning, guided imagery, talking to a supportive person, lying on warm sheets, and calling "time out" when pain gets to an overwhelming level can all help to minimize your discomfort. Asking your wound team to explain exactly what they are doing can also reduce your pain. Your wound team can also refer you to the appropriate specialists to help you further with pain management without medications.

Using Medications to Treat Pain

The most common approach to treating pain is the use of medications. Usually the goal of pain management in a chronic wound is to decrease the pain to a tolerable level, since completely eliminating the pain may not be possible. As individual experiences of pain and ability to tolerate specific medications vary, medication regimens must be adapted to the specific person. Pain medications can be used in older people (see below), but the dose should be started lower and should be increased at a slower rate.

The World Health Organization classifies pain into three categories: mild, moderate, or severe. They suggest that mild pain should be treated with mild analgesics (such as acetaminophen at the proper dosage), while moderate to severe pain may need stronger medications such as opioids.

Usually, taking medications regularly (around-the-clock), rather than just when the pain gets severe, is most effective. It is easier to prevent pain with medications than to treat it once it occurs and is out of control. Taking a medication as prescribed thirty to forty-five minutes before dressing changes or debridement can be very helpful. Anti-inflammatories can be helpful, but have risks (particularly in older people), including internal bleeding and kidney failure. There is even some evidence that anti-inflammatories may impair healing. It is important to talk to your doctor and wound team about any medications you are taking, even over-the-counter medications, since interactions between your pain medications and other drugs may occur. Never start or stop a medication without talking to your doctor first.

Tell All Your Doctors About All Your Medications

If your wound team recommends or prescribes a medication, be sure to communicate this to your primary care doctor. You should also ask the wound team to inform your primary care doctor directly regarding any medication change. By having both you and the wound team be responsible for knowing your medications, there is less chance of experiencing potentially severe consequences of medication interactions.

Nerve Pain

Nerve pain, also called neuropathic pain*, can be the worst type of pain because science has not yet found good ways to treat it. Most types of pain are due to inflammation in the tissues from a specific cause, and we have good ways of treating that type of inflammation. However, damage to the nerves (for example, in the feet and lower legs) is not caused by a particular cause or trigger and is unpredictable. This type of pain often feels like a tingling, stinging, burning, stabbing, or shooting. Some people feel electric shock–like sensations. If this nerve injury continues for a long time, the nerves can become extra sensitive, so even a light touch (such as a bed sheet lying on the feet) can cause overwhelming pain.

Nerve pain is common in persons with diabetes because uncontrolled high blood sugar can cause nerve damage. Nerve pain also can occur in amputation sites because during the amputation nerves can be severed and damaged. This is why some people sense a lot of pain in the site where the limb was, even after amputation. In some cases, this "phantom limb pain" can be very severe and is felt as though the limb were still there.

Nerve pain may need treatment with specific drugs such as antidepressants (at much lower doses than when given to treat depression) or
anti-epilepsy agents (again, at different doses than for epilepsy).

Pain in Individuals with Paralysis

People with spinal cord injury may not feel the area around the wound
during debridement, but may experience autonomic dysreflexia, which
can cause spasms, sweating, and skyrocketing blood pressure. Your
wound doctor may inject local anesthetics around the wound during
debridement to help you avoid autonomic dysreflexia.

Older People and Pain

Some myths about pain that many older people and their families may
have are shown in Table 8, with the right answer in the column next
to them.

The most important thing is to talk to your wound team, and get answers to any concerns you may have regarding pain and its treatment.

Pain in Individuals Who Cannot Verbally Communicate

A person with severe dementia or who cannot speak (such as after a severe stroke) may not be able to tell you in words that they have pain.
But they have other ways of communicating. The best thing to do in
these situations is to watch your loved one for evidence of pain-related
behaviors (such as wincing or groaning) during movement or dressing changes. Agitated behaviors, decreased appetite, sleep problems,
and functional changes can all be ways that your loved one is exhibit-
ing a pain response. Rapidly worsening confusion can also be evidence
of pain.

Even people with mild or moderate memory problems can tell you
how severe their pain is. When asking questions about pain, do so in
a "yes-or-no" format. No one is sure whether dementia affects how
pain is felt, but certainly if someone is demented and has one or more
conditions associated with significant pain (such as chronic wounds,

Table 8: Myths and Realities About Older Adults and Pain

Myth	Reality
Pain is inevitable as you get older	Pain is not normal as we age
Pain cannot be treated	Pain can often can be treated very well, even in older adults
The tests needed to diagnose the pain are going to be more painful than the pain itself	Most tests needed to diagnose pain in your wound are noninvasive and not painful
The medications needed to treat the pain are going to cause terrible side effects, such as confusion or constipation	Older people are at higher risk of developing side effects from some pain medications. This is why it is important that your doctor know how to treat older people (a geriatric specialist* can help). If medications are started at a lower dose and the dose is increased slowly, pain in an older person can be treated very well with little or no side effects.
It is easy to get addicted to pain medications	Research shows that if you take pain medications as prescribed for medical reasons, it is unlikely you will get addicted. Often, the pain medications are given for a short period of time. Sometimes, you need higher doses after a while, because you become tolerant of a certain dose . . . but this is not because of addiction.

arthritis, cancer, or poor blood flow), always be on the lookout for signs of pain or discomfort.

Pain is not just a bad feeling; it has many other negative effects. It makes dressing changes, which are an important part of wound healing, difficult to bear. It has a big impact on your quality of life and it can lead to depression. Pain itself can lead to delayed wound healing. Pain is an important gauge for you and increased pain may mean you are developing an infection. Pain is something you should not bear silently. Be sure to talk about it with your wound team.

We had been seeing Mrs. V for months in our clinic. She always was very stoic and never told us she was having pain, even though we always asked her if she did. Over time, her wound began to worsen. Finally, she admitted to us that she was not able to change the dressings as frequently as we had recommended because it hurt too much. Once we understood this, we switched Mrs. V to a special nonstick wound dressing, and also started her on a pain medication pill. We gradually increased the dose of pain medication over several weeks, and made sure she was not having any side effects. Once she was able to change the dressings as recommended, her wound finally started to heal and she needed less pain medication.

35
Skin Problems That Coexist with Wounds

Mrs. T is a fifty-six-year-old woman who works as a personal support aide and is very friendly and caring. Her mother, whose health is deteriorating, lives with her, and she spends much of her free time, day and night, caring for her mother.

Mrs. T had been seeing us for nearly a year because of her venous leg ulcers. There are many factors that slow the healing of her leg wounds: she stands a lot in her job, is obese, not getting adequate sleep, and, understandably, is finding life quite stressful. Over the past few visits to our clinic, her legs have become very red and itchy.

In this chapter, we will discuss some common issues that occur in or around wounds. In order to take care of your skin, you need to inspect it regularly to make sure there is no skin irritation or breakdown. You also need to clean and moisturize your skin properly. We'll show you how you can do this the right way.

Inspecting Your Skin

If you are at risk for developing pressure ulcers (see Chapter 5) it is important to routinely inspect your skin at least once daily. Redness that occurs after pressure is removed is commonly the first sign of a pressure ulcer. Check for any areas of redness—it might be necessary to ask a family member or health-care worker to help you with this if you have impaired vision or if you cannot easily see certain areas (such as your back or buttocks).

Cleaning Your Skin

Good skin hygiene will help lower the chances that you will develop skin irritation, infection, and even wounds. Usually, cleaning your skin with a gentle, fragrance-free soap (such as Dove) or other gentle cleanser (such as Cetaphil) and warm water is enough to ensure good skin hygiene. Use a soft cloth to pat, rather than rub, your skin dry. Avoid scrubbing or using harsh cleaning agents.

Older people (over the age of sixty-five years) do not need to bathe daily and in fact can develop dry, itchy skin if they do. Bathing or showering once or twice per week may be sufficient for many older people.

Protecting the Skin Around Your Wound

When the skin around a wound becomes waterlogged, it usually becomes white and fragile. This fragile skin is more likely to become irritated or infected than normal, healthy skin. Skin protection is particularly important if you are incontinent of urine, stool, or both, as both of these may contribute to wound worsening. So it is important not just to take care of the wound, but the skin around the wound.

There are many products available to protect the area around your wound. Some examples are zinc oxide (like what you would put on a baby's bottom to protect it) or petroleum jelly. Speak to your wound care team for more suggestions.

Dry Skin

Dry skin is one of the biggest risk factors for developing chronic wounds, particularly pressure ulcers. Skin becomes dry, flaky, and more fragile when it loses moisture. When it becomes dry and fragile, it is more prone to developing a wound. It is therefore very important to keep your skin moisturized—but you need to use the right type of moisturizers, otherwise your skin could end up becoming irritated, allergic, or worse.

Remember that more expensive is not necessarily better when it comes to moisturizers. Many inexpensive moisturizers at your neighborhood drugstore can work very well (Figure 30). Some examples of

Which moisturizer should I use?

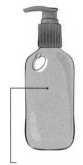
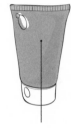
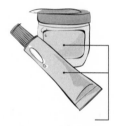

Lotions have the highest water content, which is why lotions feel cool as they are applied. They also evaporate faster than any other type of moisturizer; consequently, they must be applied more often.

Creams are a combination of oil and water. They don't have to be applied as often as lotions, but three or four applications per day may sometimes still be necessary. Creams are better for preventing moisture loss due to evaporation than for treating dry skin once it has occurred.

Ointments are prepared with placing water in oil (usually petroleum). They are the longest-lasting form of moisturizer.

Figure 30: Many inexpensive moisturizers at your neighborhood drugstore can work very well.

good brands of moisturizers for many people are Cetaphil, Neutrogena, and Lubriderm.

Moisturizers are usually grouped into one of three categories: lotions, creams, and ointments. Each of these look and feel different, and have their own advantages and disadvantages.

Lotions

Lotions have the highest water content, which is why lotions feel cool as they are applied to your skin. Lotions evaporate faster than any other type of moisturizer; as a result, you need to apply them more often. The best lotions for use on dry skin are fragrance-free and hypoallergenic.

Creams

Creams are a combination of oil and water. Creams don't have to be applied as often as lotions, but you still may need to apply them up to three or four times a day. Creams are better than lotions for preventing dry skin than for treating dry skin once it has occurred.

Ointments

Ointments are mostly oil (usually petroleum), but also include water. Ointments are the longest-lasting form of moisturizer.

Whatever type of moisturizer you use, make sure that it doesn't contain any of the ingredients listed in the "Use with Caution!" box. As always, speak to your wound team if you have any concerns or questions.

Skin Irritation from Incontinence

There needs to be a balance in how moist your skin is: if your skin is too dry, you could develop a wound. The opposite is also true: if your skin is too wet, your skin is also more likely to break down into a wound. A frequent reason that skin becomes too wet is incontinence from loss of bowel or bladder control.

Use with Caution!

Look at the ingredients of any products that you put on your skin or wound. If you have or have ever had a chronic wound, do not use products with any of the following ingredients unless you talk to your wound team first.

Lanolin
Rosin
Propylene glycol
Parabens
Lubricants
Tulle dressings
Formaldehyde
Benzocaine
Neomycin
Fragrance
Rubber (including latex)
Certain topical anesthetic creams
Bacitracin

What causes incontinence? It can occur for the first time when you are hospitalized. It may be caused by some medications or a delay in getting to the toilet in time. It may be hard for you emotionally to ask for help getting to the toilet. Many causes of incontinence can be treated without medication—a referral to a geriatric medicine specialist may help. Simple things like no fluids (except with medications) after 6 p.m., reducing your caffeine intake, switching to herbal tea from regular tea, and starting to go to the toilet regularly (for example, at least every four hours) during the day to empty your bladder, can all make a profound impact on decreasing the frequency of incontinence.

If you have had an episode of incontinence, clean the area with a mild skin cleanser (see "Cleaning Your Skin" above), then rinse and pat the skin dry. Applying a moisture barrier ointment can help to protect your skin the next time incontinence occurs, by keeping away the irritating agents in urine or stool. Your wound care team can advise you on what products may be right to protect your skin.

Allergic Skin Reactions

People with chronic wounds, especially on the legs, can be almost ten times as likely as people who have not had chronic wounds to develop allergies from products they put on their skin.

If you are using a product on your skin and your skin in that area becomes itchy, red, very dry, and/or swollen, you may be allergic to that product. You should discontinue using it until you speak to your doctor or wound care team. If you don't discontinue using it, the rash can eventually spread all over your body. These allergic skin rashes can usually be treated easily, especially if caught early. Call your wound team as soon as you notice any skin irritation that you suspect may be a skin allergy.

Itching—It's Driving Me Crazy!

Many people say that the itch is the worst part about having a wound. But it is usually quite easy to treat, so talk to your wound team. Itching around a chronic wound is most often due to dry skin (discussed above), and allergic reaction to a topical agent (discussed above), or irritated skin due to drainage from the wound.

A Fungus Among Us

Fungus usually makes its home in moist areas of the body where skin surfaces meet: between the toes, in the genital area, and under the breasts.

Fungal skin infections can cause a bright red rash, sometimes with some skin breakdown. Small pimple-like bumps may appear at the

Risk Factors for a Fungal Skin Infection

- Hot, humid conditions
- Tight synthetic undergarments
- Poor hygiene
- Inflammatory skin disease such as psoriasis
- Antibiotics (antibiotics kill the bacteria that normally live in the body, allowing fungi to grow unchecked)
- Corticosteroid medication (by mouth or by inhaler)
- Suppressed immune system (for example, after organ transplant)
- Pregnancy
- Obesity (because of excess skin folds)
- Diabetes

edges of the rash. The rash may burn or itch a lot. Diaper rash in babies is often a type of fungal infection.

Fungal infections can also occur in your nails, especially if you have diabetes. If your nails turn white or yellow, this may indicate a fungal infection. These nail infections don't often spread. They can be hard to treat, and the medications used to treat them are often expensive in addition to causing side effects, so it is often preferable to not treat them. If you are concerned about your fingernails or a possible infection, discuss it with your health-care provider.

If you have a rash that your doctor thinks may be caused by a fungus, he or she can usually confirm the diagnosis by scraping off a small amount of skin and having it examined under a microscope.

Fungal skin infections are usually very easily cured with special creams. You can buy many antifungal creams without a prescription (though if you are prone to developing wounds, you should see your

Athlete's Foot

Athlete's foot (medical term: tinea pedis) is a common fungal infection that may spread from person to person in communal showers or other moist areas where people walk barefoot. The fungus causes scaling and peeling of skin, or redness and itching. Usually, athlete's foot occurs in the moist areas between the toes, or may even involve the entire sole of the foot. Sometimes the toenails can get infected. The fungus may cause your skin to crack, which can allow bacteria to enter and cause a more serious infection. This is why it is important to treat athlete's foot early, especially in older people, people with diabetes, and those with poor blood flow.

wound team first to make sure that what you have is a fungal infection and not something else). Antifungal powders usually do not work as well as the creams. The cream is usually applied once or twice daily for seven to ten days until the rash has completely disappeared. If you stop using the cream too soon, the infection may not be completely treated and the rash will come back. Keeping the skin dry also helps clear up the infection and prevents it from returning.

If you have a more serious fungal skin infection, one that doesn't go away with a cream, or if you have a fungal scalp or nail infection, your doctor may prescribe an antifungal drug to be taken by mouth. This drug often needs to be taken for a long time and can have serious side effects in certain people.

Scars

After a chronic wound has healed, you are often left with a scar. Scar formation is a natural part of the healing process after injury. A scar isn't so bad if it's small or in a location that's easy to conceal. However, many chronic wounds are large and so may leave an extensive scar. Unfortunately, the scar will probably never completely go away, but the good news is that there are things you can do to reduce its size and improve its appearance. And the best news is—the wound healed!

Just as everyone heals differently, everyone scars differently, too. The larger and deeper the wound, the larger the scar is likely to be. Your age, genes, and your skin color all affect how you scar. The older you are, if your parents tended to scar and if you have darker skin, you are more likely to have a scar as a result of a wound or other injury. African Americans are more likely to develop keloid scars (see Chapter 25 for more information on keloid scars).

If you have suffered from a burn injury in the areas of your joints, you may have tightening of the skin that can affect your ability to move. In these cases, surgery can sometimes help. You can sometimes receive a skin graft, where the surgeon removes skin from another area of your body and applies it to the scarred area. Physiotherapy and occupational therapy can also help you to increase your range of motion and ability to move.

Scar treatments may include over-the-counter or prescription creams (which may not work that well to reduce scars), steroid injections into the scar, silicone gel sheetings, skin grafts, dermabrasion, or laser surgery. It is best that you wait at least a year before making a decision about scar treatment. Many scars fade and become less noticeable over time.

We were quite worried when we saw how red Mrs. T's legs were under her compression bandaging. As we discussed in this chapter, people with chronic wounds can easily develop sensitivities to some of the products and dressings. One of the products that people can easily become sensitive to is latex, which is found in many compression dressings. Changing standard compression bandaging to latex-free dressings can help resolve leg redness.

Mrs. T switched to latex-free compression, and we prescribed a steroid cream for her to put on her red skin to decrease the inflammation and itching. We also sent her to a dermatologist for patch testing to confirm our suspicion of a latex allergy, which it did. A few weeks after her compression was changed, Mrs. T's legs became less red and the itching had completely stopped. Her quality of life greatly improved.

36
Emotional Aspects of Wound Healing
When the Wound Is More than Skin Deep

Chronic wounds affect your quality of life and can take an emotional toll on you and your family. There is a wide range of emotional reactions you may have to your situation. It is common to feel frustrated, anxious, angry, or depressed (sometimes all at the same time). You can be sure that they are all normal feelings commonly experienced by people with wounds.

In this chapter, we help you to identify when you are having these feelings and help you decide when to seek help. We offer suggestions on how you can begin to heal emotionally so that you can heal physically.

Common Emotional Responses to Chronic Wounds

This Is Embarrassing!

When your wound is heavily draining and there is an odor, it can make you uncomfortable to be around other people. You may not even want your friends and family to be around you because you know the smell will bother them. These feelings of embarrassment about your wound may make you decide not to attend social functions that you would otherwise really enjoy. Your wound may become a decisive factor on whether you go out with your friends, to church, weddings or other special occasions. This can make you feel very isolated.

I Don't Know Who I Am Anymore

Having a wound may affect not only the decisions you make but how you live your life. You might not be able to participate in the same work activities that you used to before your wound; you may even have to give up working if it is slowing the healing of your wound. You may not be able to attend your children's events because of scheduled dressing changes. It may be tricky to plan trips with your family or friends because of doctors' visits or dressing change issues. You might not be able to be the same parent or spouse or caregiver that you used to be before your wound.

It is important to focus on the things you *can* do for your friends and family (which is easier said than done), rather on the things you cannot, and find ways to problem-solve within these new limits. A qualified therapist, particularly one experienced in dealing with people with chronic illness, can be invaluable in helping you to do this.

Changes in Your Sex Life

A wound may change many aspects of your relationship with your partner. You may have become your partner's caregiver and care for his or her wound (or vice versa). This may cause the relationship to become more like a patient-caregiver relationship rather than an intimate one. Having the wound may embarrass you during intimate situations. All of this can be very challenging and may lead to depression if not dealt with. It is important to develop and maintain a strong ongoing communication regarding physical intimacy with your partner so that these issues can be addressed as they arise.

Stress, Depression, and Anxiety

The way you feel emotionally directly impacts how you heal physically. The mind and body are connected very deeply. When you feel stressed, you are more likely to experience wound pain and prolonged wound healing. It can be a vicious cycle, so it is important to stop the cycle. People who are very anxious report more severe pain and have higher cortisol (a stress hormone in the blood) and blood pressure. Stress and depression have also been linked to changes in the immune system. What this means is that if you feel constantly stressed and depressed, you may be more prone to wound infection. In fact, one study found that wound healing was slower in people who were part of a "hostile marriage."

Depression is common in people with many chronic illnesses, and chronic wounds are no different. It can be depressing to have pain and not be able to participate in activities or perform your normal work. Many people with chronic wounds become very anxious, and not just about their wound care. Having a nonhealing wound for a long period of time can make you feel on edge about almost everything in your life.

What Can I Do to Feel Better?

If you are feeling stressed, anxious, or depressed, it is important that you talk to your wound team—they can help. All of these are common responses to a frustrating problem. There are effective treatments for

A Closer Look at Depression and Anxiety in People with Wounds

In one study of 190 people with chronic venous ulcers, 52 (27 percent) people were depressed while 50 (26 percent) were anxious.

The two symptoms that appeared to be most associated with anxiety and depression were *pain* in the wound and *odor* from the wound. So if your wound is not healing, it is important to talk to your wound team about managing any pain and odor, as these two things are most likely to cause you distress.

anxiety and depression, which include counseling and medications. Depending on your specific situation, there may be a support group available, where you could talk to others with wounds and also find out about other resources you may not otherwise know about.

It may also help you to make a list of things that help make you feel better if you begin to feel overwhelmed. Make this list when you are feeling good, and look at it when you are feeling stressed. Answer the following questions:

- Is there a type of music that relaxes me?
- Which friend or family members make me feel better? (Don't call anyone who will just make you feel worse!)
- What else calms my nerves? (For example, petting your cat or dog, going for a walk)

Talk to your wound team: research has shown that when health professionals explain what they are doing, or guide you in methods of relaxation, or allow you to listen to music during an uncomfortable procedure, people feel better. These same approaches would probably help ease your discomfort and pain during dressing changes and wound debridement.

Many studies show that people with chronic wounds suffer limitations of activity and mobility, more severe pain, and increased worries about their health, as well as significantly lower self-esteem. Improvements in the wound and wound care may significantly improve your quality of life and self-esteem.

Pain and Your Emotions

Six out of every ten patients with venous leg ulcers have pain with their ulcer. This is probably true for other types of chronic wounds too. Talk to your wound team about your pain, since chronic wound pain if left untreated can lead to depression. Pain is particularly important in older people, when it can cause severe impairment in the ability to live alone independently. Preventing and treating pain is discussed in Chapter 34.

Healthy Coping Strategies

Here are some recommendations for coping with the emotional weight of having a wound:

- Work with your wound team to set reasonable, specific goals for treating and managing your wound.
- Be open to learning about your condition and effective self-care.
- Use the treatments your health-care team recommends— if you don't agree with them, discuss your reasons with your team.
- Avoid denial and pessimism—be an active player in setting the course of your care.
- Don't compare yourself or your life to your prewound state—work to accept what is happening and move forward.
- Don't be afraid to discuss these emotional concerns with your wound team—they've certainly heard of these difficulties before and probably have useful suggestions. You are not alone.

It is important to ask for help; your wound team can help you with the pain or refer you to a specialist who can help. Individual reactions to pain vary. Some people feel that they have no control over the situation. Others empower themselves to learn more and become experts in their own condition, often using the Internet to access information and asking their wound team questions. Some people appear not interested in their wound—denial is their coping strategy. It is important for you to develop healthy coping strategies and empower yourself so you can manage the challenges of your wound and of your life.

37
Care for the Caregiver
Beating the Burnout

Betty and Homer are retired and are in their late seventies. They maintain a home together and love to travel. Homer has had venous ulcers on and off for years, but has otherwise been very well until recently.

Over the past year, Homer has not been able to remember things as well as he used to. He is also weaker and needs help from Betty to get dressed, go to the bathroom, and perform dressing changes on his ulcers. Betty has been able to help her husband and seemed to be coping.

The last time they came to our clinic, they came by ambulance instead of in their car. Homer was not talking very much and he seemed very weak. Betty looked very upset. When we asked how she was coping, she asked to speak with the team without her husband present. As she started talking, she burst into tears. She said she needed help to turn her husband while he was in bed to prevent pressure sores. She was also worried about him falling when she was taking him to the bathroom. He was soiling the bed and she was exhausted from changing the sheets so much. She said she was doing the best she could but she was so tired that she worried she wasn't going to be able to keep going.

The caregiver is an essential member of the patient's team and needs to be considered in every treatment decision. Approximately 22.4 million people in the United States provide some form of care to someone who is elderly, ill, or disabled. The situation is particularly challenging for those in the "sandwich generation" who are caring for aging parents and raising children at the same time. Caregiver stress is associated with increased risk of illness for the caregiver and even death.

While you may get much gratification from caring for a loved one, as a caregiver you are also responsible for someone else's physical, mental, and emotional health. How do you care for others while taking care of yourself? Too often, the answer is that the caregiver takes excellent care of their loved one, but neglects themselves. How can you keep yourself and the one you're caring for free from further injury? What is the best way to make the one you're caring for comfortable? In this chapter, we will help you find answers to these questions and more.

 Some Facts on the Enormous Demands of Caregiving

- One-quarter of adults are caring for an elderly relative (and 45 percent of this group are caring for their spouse)
- The family caregiver is usually the spouse or child (most often the eldest daughter, or daughter-in-law) who lives closest to the family member needing care.
- According to a survey by Home Instead Senior Care, 31 percent of family caregivers admit they'd like more help, and 25 percent resent other family members who don't help out more.
- The caregiver provides on average twenty-one hours of assistance a week for 4.3 years, according to a 2004 study by AARP and the National Alliance for Caregiving.

Additional Resources at the back of the book offers some resources you can contact for further assistance.

Caregivers face a variety of physical, emotional, and financial burdens that can cause caregiver stress. If caregivers are not able to take care of themselves, they can quickly develop caregiver burnout.

Physical Demands

As a caregiver, you are often required to do a number of physical tasks that can stress the body and the spirit. These may include:

- Bending over to do dressing changes
- Lifting your loved one (in and out of a bed, wheelchair, bathtub, or car)
- Turning your loved one from side to side in bed to prevent pressure sores
- Bathing
- Feeding
- Administering medications
- Cooking for your loved one as well as for yourself
- Additional shopping
- Accompanying or driving your loved one to doctor's appointments and other errands

These activities can be very exhausting, especially on top of other demands such as attending to finances, caring for your children, and working outside the home. These physical demands can be even more difficult if you have medical problems yourself.

Emotional Demands

Caring for someone who is ill or disabled can be very taxing emotionally as well. Sometimes the person you are caring for may have memory problems or dementia and cannot remember you, or has a hard time communicating with you or following commands. Your loved one may have behavioral problems such as yelling, hitting, biting, or wandering away, and may have changeable moods and emotional states. These may understandably make you feel frustrated, angry, or resentful toward your loved one.

Financial Demands

Let's face it—caring for someone can be a thankless job, and it is almost always done without pay. The National Family Caregivers Association and Family Caregiver Alliance estimate that unpaid relatives give over $306 billion worth of care a year. That is twice as much as home care workers and nurses get paid. You may be spending so much time taking care of someone else that you can no longer work outside the home and bring in a paycheck. Caring for your loved one can be expensive in other ways: many items you need are not covered by insurance, such as some wound dressings, appropriate footwear, incontinence products. This huge financial burden can make you very stressed, anxious, and depressed.

Caregiver Stress

Caregiver stress is a very real consequence of the work you do to keep your loved one well. It would probably be abnormal to not have any days when you feel stressed. We all feel stress sometimes. However, stress that doesn't get any better after a short time or is getting worse needs to be dealt with—or else it can lead to burnout.

I'm Stressed! Now What?

Remember that caregiver stress affects many people and is a normal reaction to a very difficult situation. Talk to your health-care team. They can suggest ways to reduce your stress. Ask family or friends for help so you can take a break. Taking care of yourself does not make you selfish or inattentive toward your loved one. Fifteen minutes taken to make yourself feel more relaxed might give you the energy to get you through the rest of the day. Asking for help does not make you a failure, and taking a short break can help reenergize and refresh you so that

Signs of Stress

- Feeling sad or moody
- Crying more than is normal for you
- Having low energy
- Feeling like you don't have any time for yourself anymore
- Changes in sleeping patterns (insomnia or sleeping too much)
- Changes in eating patterns (having no appetite or overeating)
- Isolating yourself from friends and family
- Losing interest in hobbies
- Feelings of anger or resentment toward the person you are caring for

All of the feelings can be normal and occur from time to time as you care for someone. However, if they are occurring regularly, you need to get help. The important thing to remember is to take care of yourself as well as your loved one. *You cannot help others if you're stressed out and sick yourself.*

you can take even better care of your loved one. If you have home care, take advantage of the times that the home health aide is there. Take a short break and if you can, get out of the house, maybe socialize with some friends or do other activities you enjoy.

Ask for Help!

You may not be able to afford private home care, but there are other resources. Try one of these resources:

- Your church, temple, mosque, or synagogue. They may have programs that offer support.
- Look into the National Family Caregiver Support Program through the U.S. Department of Health and Human Service's Administration on Aging. They can assist you in finding resources in your area. Their website can be found at www.eldercare.gov or you can call 1–800–677–1116 for more information.

You are not alone. There are organizations that know how difficult it is to care for a loved one with a chronic medical condition and offer programs to help people in your situation.

What Help Should I Ask For?

Simple help with small tasks can be a load off your mind and make you feel less isolated with your situation. It might seem like an imposition, but this gesture could pay you back by helping you recuperate some energy. Consider asking a family member, friend, or neighbor to help:

- Pick up some groceries
- Fill a prescription
- Assist you in handling a few household chores
- Keep the person you're caring for company so you can have a cup of tea, get some fresh air, or just have a bit of unstructured time

Remember: When help is offered, accept it, and delegate a specific task! If you don't balance caregiving with your own life and everyday needs, you cannot truly serve someone else—instead, you will burn out and serve neither one of you.

What You Can Do to Feel Better

First of all, know that you are not superhuman and do not feel guilty when you take time to reenergize yourself. Your mental and physical health is as important as your loved one's. The suggestions below can go a long way to making you feel better and stronger.

1. Exercise. Though you may not have time to officially "work out," you can make exercise part of everything you do. One idea is to walk around the hospital while waiting for a loved one's appointment.

2. Eat properly. You may be preparing nutritional meals for your loved one and neglecting yourself—it is important that you eat well, too.

3. Sleep. Being tired can make your day harder and makes it more difficult to manage your emotions and care for your loved one.

4. Get a massage. Massages can do wonders for your emotional and physical health, and are often at least partially reimbursed if you have a prescription from your doctor. Many massage schools also offer services at discount rates.

5. Pursue a hobby. A hobby (such as gardening, drawing, or playing the piano) can help bring you joy and even get you out of the house to socialize. It's okay to escape—your loved one wants you to enjoy your life.

6. Practice relaxation techniques. Many stress management relaxation classes are available. Often, stress management workshops are available in hospitals and health clinics. Deep muscle relaxation, visualization, and proper breathing can all be very helpful.

7. Ask for help. Don't be afraid to do this—many people, such as your neighbors, that you know may want to help but don't know what you need.

8. Join a caregivers support group. Contact your local ACS to find the nearest group. It's important to connect with people who share similar experiences.

Caregiver Burnout

Burnout occurs when you feel so overwhelmed that you are unable to care for your loved one and often unable to care for yourself. It oc-

Signs of Burnout

If stress continues without being treated, it can lead to something more severe: caregiver burnout. Here are some signs:

- You are irritable, have a short fuse, and snap at people for small things. You lose patience easily.
- You don't stay in touch with friends and activities like you used to.
- You are constantly tired and exhausted.
- You have a hard time getting to sleep or staying asleep, or sleep restlessly.
- You feel numb and apathetic and must force yourself to do routine tasks.
- Appetite changes. You eat more than you used to or don't feel like eating at all.
- Substance use. Your intake of alcohol, cigarettes, or other drugs increases.
- You feel guilty. You feel that you are not doing enough, or resent the amount of work you're doing.

curs if caregiver stress is not prevented or managed early on. If you think you are reaching the point of burnout, you need to get medical attention.

It may be that you need more help in caring for your loved one. Your health-care team can help you find resources in your community. Some examples include:

- Adult day care: These facilities offer older adults a place to socialize and participate in activities. The program may run for one half-day a week or more, and provide you a break. This may be an option if your loved one is able to safely leave home. Some adult day care programs offer transportation to and from their facilities.

- Respite care: Skilled nursing facilities (such as nursing homes or assisted living facilities) are often able to take your loved one for a period of time (for example, from a weekend to two to four weeks) in order to give you a break.
- Support groups: Support groups can be very beneficial and allow you to receive emotional and social support from others.
- Private care: If you have the money, you can hire a private aide to help, whether just for a couple of hours a day to give you a break, or for twenty-four hours a day.

If You Would Like to Help a Caregiver

When you help a caregiver, you are helping two people: the caregiver and the one he or she cares for. Your help will certainly be appreciated. If you don't know where to begin or how to help, here are some suggested things you can do that will be invaluable:

- Listen. Ask how the caregiver is doing. How is he/she coping? Be sincere, understanding, and compassionate and really listen to the caregiver's response. Don't give advice unless you are asked.
- Offer to run simple errands like getting groceries or picking up items at the drugstore.
- Give the caregiver a chance to get out of the house. Offer to stay with the care recipient while the caregiver goes out and relaxes.
- Help keep humor in their life.

Betty was overwhelmed by the challenge of caring for her husband. She was tired and felt like a failure. She hadn't realized just how sick her husband had become—it seemed to happen so fast. We sent Homer from our clinic to the emergency room because he was very ill, and his medical problems extended well beyond his wounds.

It turned out that Homer had pneumonia and stayed in the hospital for several days. During that time we were able to connect Betty with a social worker, who was able to get Betty more help in her home. While Homer was in the hospital, Betty was able to get some sleep and felt better. With this time apart from her husband, she was able to call her family and friends to tell them just how hard things had been. When her family and friends realized this, they helped Betty arrange for more support from her church. By the time Homer returned home, she had more help in place and felt like she would be able to meet the challenge of caring for her husband again.

38

Online Medical Resources

How to Separate Clever Advertising from
Effective Medicine

The Internet can be a great tool to learn more about your health and there is a lot of great information out there. The problem is that there is also a lot of misinformation on the Internet. Some of this untrustworthy information can simply be misleading or inaccurate, and other information may be downright dangerous. It can be difficult to know the difference between useful information based on good science and useless information not based on science.

The most important thing to know is that anyone can put health information on the Internet. Generally, good quality information will have the name of the author or organization (such as a university or hospital) clearly displayed on the website. Ask yourself these questions:

- What are the qualifications and experience of the author or organization? If you are going to implement any of the information you read, make sure that the information was written by a health professional who has a license to practice in his or her field.
- When was the information written? Some websites display out-of-date information.

- Is anyone profiting financially or otherwise from the information on the website? Websites run by the manufacturer of a product may be biased in favor of their product.

Where Can I Find Good Information?

It is best to look for websites that are run by an unbiased author or organization. Large nationwide associations for specific diseases (such as the American Diabetes Association), universities (which must meet academic standards and are nonprofit), hospitals, and government websites can all be helpful. See Additional Resources at the back of the book for websites related to treating chronic wounds that we have found useful.

To Blog or Not to Blog?

The Internet can be a great way to connect with other people going through the same things as you are. Chat groups and blogs can help make you feel less alone, and give you ways to cope that you might not have thought of. But beware: what works for someone else might not work for you. Be on the lookout for bad advice. Talking to your wound team about what you have read can help you decide whether the suggestions are right for you.

Be aware that if you disclose personal information on the Internet (when registering for a site or leaving a comment on a blog or in a patient forum), it may be available to nearly anyone in the world with an Internet connection. Guard your privacy if this is of concern to you.

Miracle Cures

There are many "miracle cures" for wounds on the Internet. The market for wound care products is highly profitable for the manufacturers, so some questionable treatments are available. Not all wound care products that are advertised or available are based on good science.

Some of these products are not only expensive, but also may damage your wound and prevent healing. Chances are if it sounds too good to be true, it is.

First, Talk to Your Wound Care Team

Before you try any suggestion or product you find on the Internet, talk to your wound care team about it. Print out the information and take it with you to your next clinic appointment, so your team can look at the information, fully understand what you have read, and see who is writing the information. In our clinic, some of our patients bring us ideas or suggestions we might not otherwise have thought of, that work very well. Other times, we unfortunately see people who have tried expensive remedies that have worsened their wounds. You can help avoid this if you work closely with your health-care team.

How to Find Reliable Websites

The following are a few sites that will teach you more about how to look for and read websites about your health.

> http://library.uchc.edu/departm/hnet/rbpopmed.html. This site by Healthnet: Connecticut Consumer Health Information Network, at the University of Connecticut Health System, discusses some useful tips for understanding health information.
> http://www.hon.ch/HONcode/Conduct.html. This website from the Health on the Net Foundation discusses the principles that good health websites should follow.
> http://www.fda.gov/Fdac/features/1999/699_fraud.html. This U.S. Food and Drug Administration webpage discusses how you can spot health fraud.

39

Payment and Reimbursement Issues
Who's Picking Up the Check?

Gary comes to our clinic for venous leg ulcer care. A visiting nurse has been dressing the wounds and applying three-layer compression bandaging three times a week. His ulcers are now completely healed. To prevent the ulcers from rapidly returning, we write a prescription for "three-layer compression wrapping three times a week for two weeks" because Gary still has edema that would not be reduced with stockings alone.

Gary calls our clinic the next day, stating that his insurance company will not pay for the visiting nurse to do the compression bandaging, since he no longer has an open wound. Our wound care team contacts the visiting nurse and finds that the insurance company will pay for compression wrapping of "persistent edema that is not alleviated by compression stockings." The wound care team rewrites the prescription, but this time states that the reason that we ordered it was for "persistent edema not alleviated by compression stockings." The visiting nurse is now able to continue the compression stocking visits under Gary's insurance.

Gary's situation illustrates how your wound care team can work with you and your family to optimize care. Filing the correct forms, obtaining preauthorizations, and using specific language and procedure codes are essential for receiving all the services you are entitled to under your insurance. The wound team should be accurate and precise about the wound treatment indications. The wound care team should also document all treatments and indications clearly in the chart for future reference.

You may be well aware that wound care can be expensive, and many costs may not be covered by your insurance. It is essential that you stay informed so you can advocate for coverage or reimbursement of your wound care costs.

Payment Systems

Some payment systems in the United States include Medicare, Medicaid, managed care, and private pay. Medicare is a federal insurance program for people age sixty-five and older and specific disabled people. Payment for services and products varies with the setting, such as

---

When Will Medicare Cover Wound Dressings?

Medicare covers surgical dressings for patients who:

- Need them to treat a wound caused by surgery or surgical procedures
- Need them after wound cleaning
- Have severe bedsores or ulcers

These patients must also:

- Have a prescription that is signed and dated by the prescriber
- Be enrolled in Medicare and have a supplier number

Tips for Getting the Wound Dressings You Need

- Contact your insurance company and/or prescription program to see if they have a formulary (approved list of products that are covered) of wound treatments. Bring this list with you to your appointments. Be aware that even if a treatment is "covered," you may still have to pay some portion of the cost, as a copay and/or coinsurance.
- Be flexible. If your insurance company does not cover a specific treatment recommended by your wound care team, keep in mind that there are thousands of products on the market, many of them that work just as well. Ask your wound team about alternatives.
- Be your own advocate. If your wound care team recommends an expensive treatment that you cannot afford and that your insurance company does not cover, inform your team. Let them know that you and the team need to come up with another plan to meet your needs.

acute care hospitals, skilled nursing facilities, home health care, outpatient clinics, and hospices.

Whether or not Medicare, Medicaid, or private pay insurers will reimburse you for wound care costs varies from region to region and depends on your medical conditions.

You should talk to your insurance company and your wound team to make sure that your wound doctor writes down the specific appropriate information your insurance carrier requires. Don't assume that all health professionals will understand that you may be having trouble paying for a wound treatment that is recommended to you.

You will probably have to bring up the topic. Because there are many wound products available, it is likely that your wound team can come up with a solution for you that will be reimbursed. Your wound team can also refer you to a social worker to help you find alternative payment sources.

Your living conditions also influence your ability to heal. Your wound team should take your home environment and your ability to apply and change the dressings into consideration when deciding what treatments to prescribe. They may refer you to home health care to assist you with dressing changes.

Reimbursement and Scars

If you have a scar as a result of a healed chronic wound and the scar is physically impairing you in any way, you may be able to get coverage from your insurance carrier. You can ask your doctor to write a letter detailing your particular situation, such as if you are a burn victim. He or she can also take photos to help prove your case. If you are undergoing scar treatment for cosmetic purposes, you will most likely have to pay for it all yourself. If your scars are caused from cosmetic surgery, insurance coverage for any elective surgery that is not medically necessary is likely to be very limited.

Glossary of Terms

Arterial ulcer: Also known as an ischemic ulcer. A wound that occurs due to poor arterial blood flow, usually due to atherosclerosis (hardening of the arteries).

Bedsore: A wound caused by skin being pressed against a surface, such as a bed, for a long time. Also called a *pressure ulcer*.

Biological dressings: Dressings derived from cells, skin, or other organic materials.

Body mass index (BMI): defined as weight (in kilograms) divided by height (meters)^2.

Charcot foot: Deformity of the foot due to neuropathy, usually related to diabetes mellitus; foot loses sensation, bones become misaligned, and a "rocker bottom" foot often results.

Chiropodist: A specialist in diseases of the foot and lower ankle. Unlike *podiatrists*, chiropodists do not perform surgery.

Chronic wound: Also known as a *nonhealing wound*. A wound that is not healing after three weeks of adequate treatment.

Circulation: Movement of blood through heart and blood vessels.

Collagen: Protein that is the main component of skin and tendons.

Debridement: Cleaning out and removal of nonviable or *necrotic tissue*; this is one of the most important factors in promoting healing of chronic wounds.

Dehiscence: Bursting or splitting open of a surgical wound after it has been closed up surgically.

Dermatologist: A physician who specializes in skin diseases.

Dietician: A licensed health professional who advises on food and eating from a scientific basis.

Edema: Swelling.

Elephantiasis: A condition where prolonged swelling leads to thickening of the skin, lymphatic fluid passing through the skin (see *lymphedema*), and leg swelling.

Endocrinologist: A physician who has specialized in the endocrine glands and hormone systems of the body.

Foot drop: When the foot cannot be flexed upward because there is weakness in the front leg muscles or there are impaired nerves.

Gangrene: Death and decay of body tissue, usually due to poor blood flow and/or infection.

Geriatrician (Geriatric specialist): A physician who specializes in the care of older adults (usually those over the age of sixty).

Hydrocolloid: A substance that forms a gel with water.

Infrared thermometer: A device that measures the temperature of the skin, and can help to diagnose infection or inflammation.

Ischemia: Poor arterial blood flow to body tissue, usually due to constriction or blockage of arterial blood vessels.

Ischemic ulcer: Also known as an *arterial ulcer*. A wound that occurs due to poor arterial blood flow, usually due to atherosclerosis (hardening of the arteries).

Lymphedema: The fluid that collects due to damage of the lymphatic system.

Maceration: White and boggy-looking skin that is a result of being wet for a long time.

Melanin: Substance that gives skin its color.

Monofilament: A thin piece of plastic used to touch the skin, in order to test for *neuropathy*.

Necrotic tissue: Dead body tissue. Usually removed during *debridement*.

Neuropathic pain: Pain due to injured nerves.

Neuropathy: Nerve damage, often caused by diabetes but has other causes. Neuropathy can be very painful and can feel like burning or stabbing pain.

Nonhealing wound: Also known as a *chronic wound*.

Nutritionist: A person who advises on food and eating from a scientific basis, but is not a regulated health-care professional.

Occupational therapist: A professional who has specialized in the assessment and treatment of self-care, work, and leisure skills, with the goal to maintain independence in these skills. The skills often involve the use of the hands and arms.

Orthopedic surgeon: A surgeon who has specialized in bone injuries.

Osteomyelitis: Infection of the bone.

Physical medicine and rehabilitation specialist: A physician who has specialized in the treatment of illnesses or injuries that affect how you move.

Physiotherapist: A professional who has specialized training in assessing and treating problems that relate to standing, walking, and other activities.

Plastic surgeon: A surgeon who has specialized in cosmetic and reconstructive surgery.

Podiatrist: A specialist in diseases of the foot and lower ankle who can perform surgery.

Psychiatrist: A physician who has specialized in mental disorders.

Pyoderma gangrenosum (PG): A skin condition that lends itself to frequent painful nonhealing ulcers, usually on the legs, but can occur anywhere on the body.

Skin biopsy: A surgical removal of skin in order to diagnose a disease; often done in an office setting with a topical pain killer.

Social worker: A professional skilled in assessing a person's physical and emotional needs and connecting people with services to meet those needs; they often integrate the family in decision making.

Swab: To use a cotton-tip applicator to get a sample of bacteria that may be growing in a wound.

Ulcer: A breakdown of the skin due to an accident or disease that results in a wound. Also called a *wound*.

Vascular surgeon: A surgeon who has specialized in blood vessel surgeries and procedures.

Venous stasis: Occurs when fluid stays in your legs because your veins are not working properly.

Venous ulcer: A wound that occurs due to poorly functioning veins. Also called a *venous stasis* ulcer.

Wound: An injury that results in a break of the skin, or bruising of the skin. Also called an *ulcer*.

Wound border: The edge of the wound.

Wound Cleansers and Dressings

Wound Issue	Type of Cleanser or Dressing	Examples	Keep in mind
Cleaning the wound	Saline Sterile water		
A lot of drainage	Alginates Hydrofibers Foams Absorptive dressings	Allevyn Polymem Aquacel Mesalt	
Not draining or draining very little	Hydrogels Hydrocolloid	Intrasite DuoDERM	These dressings can make the wound and surrounding skin too wet
Dry wound or scab	Hydrogel Antiseptics (if little blood flow)	Intrasite Povidone-iodine	
Infected wound	Cadexomer iodine Silver (Ag) dressings	Iodosorb/ Iodoflex Acticoat Aquacel Ag Contreet Silvasorb	
Severe odor in the wound	Activated charcoal Topical metronidazole Antibiotic creams Antiseptics		

(continues)

Wound Cleansers and Dressing (*continued*)

Painful wound	Hydrogel Nonstick dressings (e.g., soft silicone)	Mepilex	Topical anesthetics may help pain medications given by mouth or through an intravenous before dressing changes may be needed
Remove dead tissue	Collagenase Papain-urea Hydrogel	Accuzyme Santyl Panafil	
Combination dressing	Silver foam	Mepilex silver foam Aquacel Ag	
Dry skin around the wound	Moisturizers		
Swelling	Compression bandaging Compression stockings	Unna boot Sur-Press Profore ACE bandage Coban	
Failure to heal with other methods	Skin substitutes Growth factors MMP inhibitors	Regranex Apligraf Dermagraft Oasis Promogran/ Prisma	
Adjunctive therapies	Negative pressure (vacuum therapy) Hyperbaric oxygen		

The Wound Patient's Bill of Rights

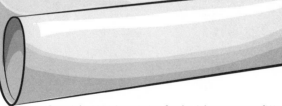

You have a right to:

- Actively participate as a member of your wound care team if you are able and willing.

- Have your wound assessed and monitored by trained health-care personnel.

- Know what wound treatment options are available to you.

- Know the benefits, risks, and side effects of your wound care treatments.

- Participate in the development of your treatment plan with your wound care team.

- Receive timely and cost-effective wound treatment.

- Have your wound treated appropriately with safe and effective products.

- Have your pain adequately controlled.

- Seek other opinions about your wound treatment plan if you so desire and consult a specialist as necessary.

- Consult other health-care professionals for advice about diet, exercise, therapy, or products.

Copyright 2006 Association for the Advancement of Wound Care (AAWC)

Copyright AAWC. Reprinted with permission from the Association for the Advancement of Wound Care. www.aawconline.org

Additional Resources

For People with All Types of Chronic Wounds

http://www.healingwell.com/
> A website devoted to living with chronic disease. This website has a forum where people can discuss problems and management strategies. It also has an article discussing different aspects of living with chronic disease.

http://www.informedhealthonline.org/index.235.en.html
> A website that describes what goes wrong in the wound that does not heal.

CLEVELAND CLINIC

http://www.clevelandclinic.org/heartcenter/pub/guide/disease/vascular/legfootulcer.htm
> Provides an overview of venous stasis ulcers, arterial ulcers, and diabetic foot ulcers in everyday language.

EUROPEAN WOUND MANAGEMENT ASSOCIATION
http://www.ewma.org/
> Information on wounds; produces guidelines for treating different chronic wounds.

CANADIAN ASSOCIATION OF WOUND CARE
http://www.cawc.net/open/library/clinical/clinical_res.html

CAWC created formal guidelines for the treatment of pressure ulcers, diabetic foot wounds, and venous leg ulcers.

For People with Diabetes Mellitus

http://organizedwisdom.com/Diabetic_Foot_Infection
Links to articles in laymen's language about diabetic foot ulcers and how they are treated.

http://www.patient.co.uk/showdoc/27000145/
Practical foot care advice for diabetics.

Special Issues

PAIN CONCERN
http://www.painconcern.org.uk/pages/page78.php
Discusses pain management in chronic wounds.

WORLD UNION OF WOUND HEALING SOCIETIES
http://www.wuwhs.org/general_publications.php
Addresses different topics such as managing pain and controlling drainage from your wound in many languages.

http://www.health.vic.gov.au/qualitycouncil/pub/improve/pupps.htm
Two patient information pamphlets on pressure ulcers.

ROYAL ADELAIDE HOSPITAL HYPERBARIC CLINIC
http://www.rah.sa.gov.au/hyperbaric/patient_info.php
Summarizes hyperbaric oxygen therapy.

WOUND CARE INFORMATION NETWORK
www.medicaledu.com/wndguide.htm
Describes the history as well as the benefits and disadvantages of maggot therapy.

For People with Amputations

AMPUTEE COALITION OF AMERICA
www.amputee-coalition.org

For People with Spinal Cord Injuries (SCI)

Pressure Ulcer Prevention and Treatment Following Spinal Cord Injury: A Clinical Practice Guideline for Health-Care Professionals
http://www.pva.org/site/DocServer/PU.pdf?docID=688
    National SCI prevention and treatment of pressure ulcer guidelines.

UNIVERSITY OF MICHIGAN HEALTH SYSTEM MODEL SPINAL
CORD INJURY CARE SYSTEM
www.med.umich.edu/opm/newspage/2002/spineexercise.htm
    Information on a study conducted by Dr. William Scelza, who
    has a spinal cord injury and is active in wheelchair basketball.

NATIONAL CENTER ON PHYSICAL ACTIVITY AND DISABILITY
www.ncpad.org/disability/fact_sheet.php?sheet=130
    Information on spinal cord injury and exercise.

www.ncpad.org/disability/fact_sheet.php?sheet=118
    An article entitled "No More Sores: Preventing Pressure Sores
    for People with SCI"

For Caregivers

CAREGIVER MEDIA GROUP
www.caregiver911.com, www.caregiver.com
    Website for Caregiver Media Group, which also produces a
    magazine and conferences on caregiving.

NATIONAL FAMILY CAREGIVERS ASSOCIATION
www.nfcacares.org, http://www.thefamilycaregiver.org

There are numerous books for caregivers available. Here are just a few:

American Medical Association Guide to Home Caregiving. New York: Wiley, 2001.

Chicken Soup for the Caregiver's Soul: Stories to Inspire Caregivers in the Home, the Community, and the World by Jack Canfield, Mark Victor Hansen, and LeAnn Thieman. Foreword by Rosalynn Carter. Deerfield Beach, Fla.: HCI, 2004.

The Fearless Caregiver: How to Get the Best Care for Your Loved One and Still Have a Life of Your Own by Gary Barg. Herndon, Va.: Capital Books, 2003.

References

Association for the Advancement of Wound Care. Wound Patient's Bill of Rights. http://www.aawcone.org/pdf/BillofRights07_06.pdf.

Bethell, E. Wound care for patients with darkly pigmented skin. *Nursing Standard* 2005; 20 (4): 41–49.

Cowan, S.M., R. D. Wallace, A. Marx, et al. Plastic surgery after loss of massive excess weight. In M. Dietel and S. M. Cowan, editors, *Update: Surgery for the Morbidly Obese Patient.* Toronto: FD Communications, 2000: 262–91.

Davidson J., and C. Callery. Care of the obesity surgery patient requiring immediate-level care or intensive care. *Obes Surg* 2001; 11: 93–97.

DeRuiter, H. P., E. Meitteunen, and K. Sauder. Improving safety for caregivers through collaborative practice. *Journal of Healthcare Safety, Compliance, and Infection Control* 2001; 5 (2): 61–64.

European Wound Management Association (EWMA). Position document: Hard-to-Heal wounds: a holistic approach. London: MEP Ltd, 2008.

Fox, H. R. Discrimination: Alive and well in the United States. *Obes Surg* 1995; 5: 21.

Freiberg, A. Plastic surgery after massive weight loss. In: M. Dietel, editor, *Update: Surgery for the Morbidly Obese Patient.* Toronto: FD Communications, 1998.

Gallagher, S. Meeting the needs of the obese patient. *Am J Nurs* 1996; 96 (8): 1s–12s.

———. Morbid obesity: A chronic disease with an impact on wounds and related problems. *Ostomy Wound Manage* 1997; 43 (5): 18–27.

———. Caring for obese patients. *Nursing* 1998; 98 (3): 32HN1–32HN5.

———. Restructuring the therapeutic environment to promote care and safety for the obese patient. *J Wound Ostomy Continence Nurs* 1999; 26: 292–97.

———. Tailoring care for the obese patient. *RN* 1999; 62 (5): 43–50.

———. Panniculectomy, documentation, reimbursement and the WOC nurse. *J Wound Ostomy Continence Nurs* 2003; 30 (2): 72–77.

———. Taking the weight off with bariatric surgery. *Nursing* 2004; 34 (3): 58–64.

Gustafson, N. J. *Managing Obesity and Eating Disorders.* Brockton, Mass.: Western Schools Press, 1997.

Harris Interactive. More than one in three U.S. adults never get a second opinion for a medical diagnosis. http://www.harrisinteractive.com/news/newsletters/clientnews/2006_Wxxi.pdf. Accessed March 30, 2008.

Jones J., W. Barr, J. Robinson, and C. Carlisle. Depression in patients with chronic venous ulceration. *Brit J Nursing,* 2006; 15 (11 Suppl 08): S17–S23.

Kean, D. P. Chronic wound healing and chronic wound management. In D. L. Krasner, G. T. Rodeheaver, and R. G. Sibbald, editors, *Chronic Wound Care: A Clinical Source Book for Healthcare Professionals.* 4th ed. Malvern, Pa.: HMP Communication, 2007: 11–24.

Kral, J. G., R. J. Strauss, and L. Wise. Perioperative risk management in obese patients. In M. Deitel, editor, *Update: Surgery for the Morbidly Obese Patient.* North York: FD Communications, 2000: 238–61.

Krasner, D. L. Managing wound pain in patients with vacuum-assisted closure devices. *Ostomy Wound Manage* 2002; 48 (5).

Kuczmarski, R. J., K. M. Fiegel, S. M. Campbell, et al. Increasing prevalence of overweight among U.S. adults: The National Health and Nutrition Examination Surveys, 1960 to 1991. *JAMA* 1994; 272: 205–11.

Lindstrom, W. So you want your insurance to cover your obesity surgery? Center for Law and Advocacy. Available at: http://www.obesitylaw.com/insurancearticle.htm. Accessed April 1, 2004.

Maiman, L. A., V. L. Wang, M. H. Becker, et al. Attitudes toward obesity and the obese among professionals. *J Am Diet Assoc* 1992; 74: 331–36.

Staffieri, J. R. A study of social stereotype of body image in children. *J Pers Soc Psychol* 1967; 7: 101–4.

Thone, R. R. *Fat: A Fate Worse than Death.* New York: Harrington Park Press, 1997.

Troia, C. Promoting positive outcomes in the obese patient. *Plast Surg Nurs* 2002; 22 (1): 10–18.

Index

Page numbers in *italics* indicate graphics.